THE
SEX ISSUE

THE
SEX
ISSUE

EVERYTHING YOU'VE ALWAYS WANTED TO KNOW ABOUT
SEXUALITY, SEDUCTION, AND DESIRE

BY THE EDITORS OF GOOP
foreword by Gwyneth Paltrow

GRAND CENTRAL

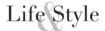

NEW YORK · BOSTON

Grand Central Life & Style
Hachette Book Group
1290 Avenue of the Americas, New York, NY 10104
grandcentrallifeandstyle.com
twitter.com/grandcentralpub

First Hardcover Edition: May 2018

Grand Central Life & Style is an imprint of Grand Central Publishing.
The Grand Central Life & Style name and logo are trademarks of Hachette Book Group, Inc.

The publisher is not responsible for websites (or their content) that are not owned by the publisher.

The Hachette Speakers Bureau provides a wide range of authors for speaking events. To find out more, go to www.hachettespeakersbureau.com or call (866) 376-6591.

Print book interior design by Fearn Cutler de Vicq.

Library of Congress Cataloging-in-Publication Data

Names: Goop, Inc., editor.
Title: The sex issue : everything you've always wanted to know about sexuality, seduction, and desire / by The editors of GOOP ; foreword by Gwyneth Paltrow.
Description: First Edition. | New York : Grand Central Life & Style, 2018.
Identifiers: LCCN 2017052345| ISBN 9781538729441 (hardback) | ISBN 9781549168499 (audio download) | ISBN 9781538729434 (ebook)
Subjects: LCSH: Sex. | Sex instruction. | BISAC: SELF-HELP / Sexual Instruction. | HEALTH & FITNESS / Women's Health. | HEALTH & FITNESS / Sexuality. | REFERENCE / Handbooks & Manuals.
Classification: LCC HQ21 .S4712 2018 | DDC 306.7—dc23
LC record available at https://lccn.loc.gov/2017052345

ISBNs: 978-1-5387-2944-1 (hardcover); 978-1-5387-2943-4 (ebook); 978-1-5491-6849-9 (audiobook, downloadable)

Printed in the United States of America

LSC-C

10 9 8 7 6 5 4 3 2 1

To our readers,

who have asked us questions about sex

we didn't know the answers to, and

who have gone on the journey with us to

find them.

contents

foreword

BY GWYNETH PALTROW

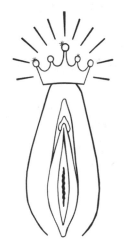

Most days lately, it feels like we're living in the midst of a seismic shift in gender issues—the feminine is really (finally) on the rise. But with every step forward, there always seems to be a pushback. When women want to ask questions that are deemed uncomfortable or impolite or out of their jurisdiction (for whatever reason), they are silenced in a myriad of ways, both blatant and subtle. The message we hear too often, whether implicit or not, is: *Stay in your lane.*

And sex is the great hot-button issue. While this is not surprising, it has been eye-opening for all of us at GOOP to see how triggering conversations around women's pleasure and sexual health can be for so many. No content we've published on the site has incited such a visceral reaction from readers (on all sides) as interviews with sexuality experts and first-person accounts of women's own experiences of their sexuality. Women talking about sex, about what they like and don't like, what they are getting and not getting in their intimate relationships, the toll of sexual trauma and how they heal—has a tendency to make people (both men and other women) extraordinarily self-conscious and uneasy.

Which isn't to say that men have it easy in the realm of intimacy. There are plenty of ways that men are silenced in relationships, and there are arguably fewer places today for men to have certain conversations around sexuality—namely those exploring vulnerability. Vulnerability is not something we as a culture do a good job of allowing boys and men to own.

The idea behind this book was to create a safe space where questions of sexuality could be explored for everyone—women, men, heterosexual, homosexual, in a relationship, single, young, experienced. It's never too late, or too early for that matter, to get comfortable with your own desires. We're fortunate at GOOP to work with a circle of thought leaders who empower us to ask questions—and who accepted our sex laundry list: everything we and readers have always wondered about seduction, attraction, dating, fantasy, orgasm, hormones, sexual power, and so on. Interspersed with the personal stories of GOOP staffers, this book is the culmination of those conversations we've had with psychotherapists, psychologists, researchers, doctors, healers, and other sex gurus. Whether tantra or BDSM or threesomes or vanilla are your thing will never be the point; knowing yourself, all your options, and how to ask for and pursue what feels good to you, is. The perspectives of bright minds included here help us, at GOOP, get there. We hope they'll support you as you look inward, too, while illuminating what's out there.

Our other hope is that this book will create more conversations off the page and be a part of destigmatizing pleasure for good. In this moment in time, there's a collective opportunity to do away with the dangerous notion that women shouldn't be completely comfortable talking about their sexuality—or that anyone should be shamed for asking questions.

In the meantime, let's keep sharing our experiences—here are ours.

Love,

GP

PART ONE

Seduction

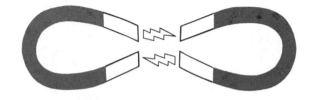

The clichés surrounding the word "seduction" tend to involve a lot of smoke and mirrors: vamping, dressing up, mind games, plotting, and consulting with trusted third parties. While all those aspects certainly have a role in sex and seduction, the experts we've assembled here tell a different, less striving, yet infinitely more powerful story.

Whether the seduction in question involves swiping right and hoping for the best, or trying to create new patterns and deepen intimacy with a long-beloved partner, seduction resides within us—in our attitudes, in our intentions, and, most of all, in our feelings about ourselves. Trying to push past that crucial grounding toward the more surface-level markers of seduction defeats the purpose. Seduction is about slowing down, feeling your power, and only then turning your focus, energy, and endless charm toward a deeply appealing other.

CHAPTER 1

what creates attraction

W hile there is undeniably an art to relationships, there also seems to be something of a science when it comes to what draws you to a particular person and vice versa. Interpersonal attraction is a research interest of Eli Finkel, a professor who holds appointments in the Department of Psychology and the Kellogg School of Management at Northwestern University. Finkel, who is also the author of *The All-or-Nothing Marriage* and the director of Northwestern's Relationships and Motivation Lab (RAMLAB), reports that physical attractiveness is the greatest predictor of initial attraction (not likely to surprise many), but that its significance decreases with time. Also important when it comes to lighting and sustaining the spark: the sense that the other person likes you uniquely (and doesn't like everyone); and avoiding the self-fulfilling prophecy trap. More from Finkel:

Decoding the Spark

ELI FINKEL, PHD

What's the difference between general attraction and sexual attraction?

Sexual attraction is a special case of general attraction. Attraction refers to the tendency to be drawn to another person, and there are many motivations for it. We might want to have fun at the pub, care for somebody who's suffering, or seek reassurance—and, of course, we might want to have sex. Psychologist Robert Sternberg argues that love consists of three components: (1) intimacy; (2) commitment; and (3) passion. From this perspective, nonsexual attraction consists of intimacy and commitment (like we might have with our mothers or our best friends), whereas sexual attraction must have passion. What's interesting is that the individual experiencing such passion might or might not also experience intimacy and/or commitment, as in cases of infatuation. Passion plays out quite differently when it's accompanied by intimacy, commitment, or both.

How important is physical attractiveness in initial attraction?

For better or for worse, however, the importance of physical attractiveness declines over time, as does the amount of agreement about who is, versus who is not, attractive.

Physical attractiveness is the single most important predictor of initial attraction. Intelligence and personality pale by comparison. For better or for worse, however, the importance of physical attractiveness declines over time, as does the amount of agreement about who is, versus who is not, attractive.

In one study, which I conducted

with Lucy Hunt and Paul Eastwick, married people who became romantically involved soon after first meeting tended to have similar levels of physical attractiveness, but people who knew each other for a while before becoming romantically involved didn't show this effect. In other words, a hot person is more likely to end up with a hot partner if they start dating shortly after meeting each other. But, if the couple gets to know each other before starting to date, this goes out the window: A hot person is just as likely to end up with a less hot partner in this case—because over time physical attractiveness becomes less important and the person's idea of what is attractive shifts.

Does low self-esteem interfere in this realm?

We know that people with low self-esteem often struggle to sustain high-quality relationships. The issue is that they often trigger a negative self-fulfilling prophecy—because they feel unworthy of love, they behave in ways that protect themselves from rejection, which in turn makes their partner more likely to leave the relationship. For example, relative to people with higher self-esteem, people with lower self-esteem tend to perceive ambiguous partner behavior (such as forgetting to text when his or her flight lands) as a sign that the partner doesn't really love them. Perceiving such signs increases their likelihood of self-protectively distancing themselves from the partner, including saying and doing hurtful things. The partner, unaware of why the other person is suddenly being distant and confrontational, generally becomes frustrated and disillusioned.

Can you explain the importance of reciprocity in attraction?

Perceiving that somebody is attracted to us is a major aphrodisiac, but only if we view his or her attraction as special. If he or she is attracted to almost everybody—perhaps because of low standards— we actually find that unappealing. In one study, which I conducted with Paul Eastwick, Daniel Mochon, and Dan Ariely, speed-daters were attracted to partners who uniquely liked them (liked them more than other people at the event), but they were turned off by partners who liked everybody. It seems that we can detect whether another person's liking for us is special vs. cheap. The special type is hot; the cheap type is not.

CHAPTER 2

how to assess attraction

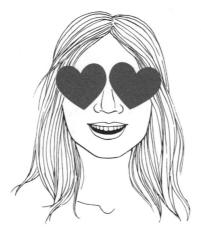

Feeling attraction and knowing when to actually act on it are not one and the same. For instance, if you're attracted to your coworker or a friend, do you go for it? How reliable is the feeling of being attracted to someone online? And why are some people, without fail, drawn to people who are so clearly not good for them? Relationship expert and life adviser Suzannah Galland has a gut check for every qualm in the dating department. Some of her advice is magic-like in that it's hard to explain why something like tossing your lingerie could help you get over an ex; but Galland is also beloved for knowing when you need the Band-Aid ripped off, and cutting right to the (blunt) point.

Rate Your Date

SUZANNAH GALLAND

***How important is immediate attraction in a potential mate? Is it a
no-go if you don't feel it?***

When it comes to attraction, I've found that first impressions are
the most reliable. Listening to our intuition, or what I call "gut hits," is key.

If someone you fancy touches your arm, it's likely butterflies will
flutter in your stomach. If you feel uncomfortable, well, that's telling
you something pretty powerful, too. If you aren't attracted to someone
when you meet them, that's generally a red flag that there is little or
no chemistry between you. There are exceptions, but the bottom line
is that it's unlikely to develop into a love relationship. I would move on
rather than invest your time in pining for something that you may or
may not feel down the road. My mantra is, "If it feels off . . . it is."

***With online dating, can you reliably judge how attracted you are to
someone before meeting them IRL?***

Online dating can be thrilling. But often, what starts out as a totally
fun prospect ends a few weeks later flat and lifeless. If this turns into a
cycle, you can quickly become exhausted.

We all have a sixth sense, whether we use it or not, and the
internet—which connects millions of us on a global scale in our cos-
mic web of consciousness—is actually a great place to use it. Think of
this sense like a tuning fork, or your GPS love guide.

Following is a tool to broaden your energy perception; in no time,
you'll be able to get a quick read on your online prospects. To keep
it simple, we'll use an energy scale of 1 to 10, with 1 being the lowest
energy level.

Take a moment and think of a person you know who has a very low,
unhappy, negative energy. (You might want to picture the first person

who broke your heart—maybe they were deceitful, irresponsible, or just let you down.) Set this up in your mind with a rating of 1. Think of level 1 as an energy sucker.

Move on now to your vision of the perfect date/partner (this depends of course on what you're looking for), someone you feel a synergistic connection with—not just in your head, but also in your body. Someone who is, say, engaging, respectful, inviting, romantic, sensual, and secure in their own person. Label this energy a 10.

For a date, you're looking for anyone above a 7—people who are exciting to you. If you accept anything less, you're allowing yourself to be pulled into a place that may drain your energy.

Now you've defined a spread in your perception from 1 to 10, which you can use to evaluate online profiles as you browse. When you do this with intention, a number will pop into your head. Try not to question it, and trust your intuition. It might seem silly—until you start getting the outcomes you want from online dating.

FROM THE GOOPASUTRA
THE LOBSTER TRAP

Think of your app profile as...a lobster trap. Some weeks the lobsters amble in, other weeks they don't; some weeks they appeal to you, some weeks they don't. In other words: no pressure, no stress. The lobster is the most sustainable seafood there is. Even if you go through a dry spell of several months—where not one single person even says hello—just know that eventually, they're going to come around.

Or, as another sage friend put it: "Treat your love life like a growing tree, and the people you date like leaves sprouting on the branches. Keep them alive and rustling but at a safe distance until you find someone you want to take more seriously."

How should we interpret attraction? When should we act on it?

If you're ever questioning how attracted you are to someone and if you should act upon your feelings, I recommend this quick mind check: Ask yourself if you would want to spend twenty minutes orally pleasuring them. This tends to tap right at the center of our sexual prowess, or sex sense.

If you're ever questioning how attracted you are to someone and if you should act upon your feelings, I recommend this quick mind check: Ask yourself if you would want to spend twenty minutes orally pleasuring them.

What if you develop an attraction to someone you already know?

We all know the excitement of striking a warm, personal spark with a friend, coworker, or even a prospective business ally. Each of us also knows how to fall in love. Here's a client example (names changed):

"It was late, everyone had left, and my colleague Cate invited me into her office. She said she wanted to ask me some advice about what to buy for her brother. We kept talking—it was an easy conversation, and it felt good being with her. There was heat, too.

"I was sitting at the edge of her desk, and leaned toward her. She moved her hand to the side of my shirt. I met her hand with mine, and she gently pulled me closer. I always knew she liked me, and I felt the same way. I knew the risks, but one thing led to another. It was clear we both wanted the same thing, to fall in love . . . or so I thought."

In this particular case, things didn't end well. There are a couple of questions worth considering if you find yourself in a similar scenario. One: Are you both looking for the same thing or have the same motivation? Is one person acting out of convenience (or being a combination of lazy and lonely), while maybe the other has stronger feelings? Is this a dalliance, a compromise, or the real deal—and are you on the same page? The other consideration to weigh concerns what is going to happen afterward, and how much any uncertainty about the future matters to you. Once you are intimate, can you both return to being just friends/ coworkers? This requires a new definition of boundaries. A casual sexual relationship can threaten the most important values of security. So, you might ask yourself: Is there just a spark or fireworks? Is it worth risking my job or this friendship? Of course, in the context of working relationships, whatever is going on isn't happening in a vacuum. There are always other dynamics at play—we should all be particularly sensitive to power dynamics in the office. If it's a colleague—or a boss—and you're walking into uncharted territory, I'd say the number one rule is to keep your power and integrity intact. Many rewarding relationships have sprung out of spending a good fifty hours a week with a colleague. Generally, these love affairs are formed over time, which helps pave the way for a more grounded love. Bottom line: As important as intuition is, it's wise to give yourself time before rushing to act on an attraction with a close friend or coworker when the stakes feel high.

If we're always attracted to people who are "wrong" for us, how do we reset?

Much like a movie that needs a rewrite, you might need to reset, reframe your own story, and change the dialogue. What image are you projecting into the world? Are you always concerned about how others see you? Often, self-esteem issues are the problem afflicting our relationships. There are many lovers out there, but attracting the right one starts with loving yourself.

How? Tell yourself one truth at least once a day that is positive—about a good thing you did, a talent you have, something that you're grateful for. Give yourself gifts. Be generous. Take the time to pamper yourself with small gestures the way you would pamper someone you love. This can be small: Rather than eating out of plastic containers, plate your meal. Wear a scent that you find romantic.

Teach yourself to be comfortable receiving small pleasures, so that you can begin to cultivate a healthy expectation that your next lover will treat you the same way—and this will in turn become more likely.

CHAPTER 3

the desire disconnect

T he road to better sex and happier relationships requires a sharp turn away from many of our deepest-held beliefs about the innate traits of men and women, says the always revelatory relationship and sexuality therapist Esther Perel. While Perel, author of *Mating in Captivity* and *The State of Affairs*, suggests that some of society's most powerful stereotypes about the differences between the genders are false, she also points toward polarities elsewhere that may seem counterintuitive initially but turn out to be surprisingly, poignantly true. Do men want sex more than women? Are women more monogamous than men? In what ways do these dynamics tend to be different or similar for same-sex couples? Perel's answers to burning questions continue to evolve the conversation around desire and sex for us all.

Who Really Gets Bored First?

ESTHER PEREL

How is desire different for men and women (or not)?

Typically, we like to think of women's desire as more discriminating. If a woman wants a man, the man can be pretty sure that it is him she wants. If a man wants a woman, she wants proof that it's her he wants.

But what we don't often admit is that women get bored with monogamy sooner than men. Research shows that men remain much more interested sexually in a partner for a longer time, with shifts being more gradual. Women tend to lose interest in a shorter amount of time and rather precipitously.

Interestingly, men in committed relationships are often much more generous. They genuinely appreciate the quality of their partner's excitement. Men in committed relationships generally talk a lot about how much they enjoy pleasing their partner. The quality of their experience often depends on the quality of *her* experience (in heterosexual relationships), seeing her enjoy it. You rarely hear a woman say: "What turns me on the most is to see him really into it." The secret of female sexuality is how narcissistic it is. What turns her on the most is to be the turn-on.

> *The secret of female sexuality is how narcissistic it is. What turns her on the most is to be the turn-on.*

It's the antidote to a woman's social world, which is so much about tending to the needs of others. In order to actually be sexual—which means to be inside her own mounting pleasures, sensations, excitement, and connection—she needs to be able to not think about others. To think about others will take her outside the sexual woman role and into the caretaking and mothering role, which are not roles that appeal to her sense of pleasure, or the selfishness that is inherent in pleasure.

Traditionally we have interpreted a woman's desire as less than a man's—we've been prone to suggest she must have less of an interest in sex. But no, it's that women become less interested in the sex they can have. Once a relationship becomes institutionalized (or formal, or legal), women often no longer feel in control. *Now she is married; here is what she is expected to do; this is what the world wants from her.* The moment a woman feels she has to do something that used to be a choice, that she felt she owned, that was hers, it becomes a duty and not a pleasure. She loses her autonomous will, which is essential to desire.

Put that same woman with a new person, in a new story, and suddenly she doesn't need a role replacement. Because she's interested in who she is, in what she's feeling, in how she's looking at herself and how she's thinking—she's turning herself on. So desire, or the lack thereof, generally doesn't have much to do with sexuality, but rather with inner criticism, lack of a sense of self-worth, lack of vitality, bad body image, you name it—because desire is to own the wanting.

What do men have a hard time talking to female partners about?

I think men have a hard time asking for support and intimacy. For example, I met a man who came from essentially nothing, in a material sense, and who has become very successful. He explained that his wife is a "type A woman who works very hard." Not the type to observe when she herself does a good job—because there is always more that she could do, or do better, in the quest for perfection. He told me about what an amazing mother she is and how much he loves her. He then discussed a year in his life that was challenging for him; he had a major business crisis, but he managed to pull through. "You know what I really wanted?" he asked me. "I just wanted my wife to put a hand on my shoulder and say, 'This is really well done, you worked so hard for this.' I needed her to be tender."

I think men want to feel admired—actually, all people want to feel admired—and to feel that women are proud of them. Many women are comfortable with self-criticism, which may also mean they're comfortable with being more vocal about what they don't like in a partner as opposed to what they appreciate. Women often need to be on the verge of losing their partners to finally start telling them everything they appreciate about them.

"I need a place where I don't have to be 'on' all the time," the man continued to tell me. "Where she can on occasion say to me: 'It's well done, good enough.'"

Why do you think some women find it hard to show compassion to their male partners?

Many women don't trust in the emotional resilience of men. They think they are superior in this realm. A woman is often afraid that if she puts her hand on her man's shoulder, he's going to break. Men are afraid of women's tensions, but women are afraid of men's meltdowns—that they will regress, suddenly going from man, to boy, to baby. Women believe that men are more fragile on some fundamental level.

Many women are also afraid that if they are compassionate with their partner, then they won't be able to lean on them. They fundamentally still want him to be strong, because that allows them to fall apart: *I need to know that you can hold me. If you're not strong, I can't let go.* This is true in sex and this is true emotionally. If or when for some reason he softens, there is a part of her that feels angry. Instead of becoming compassionate, she becomes angry.

It's like the man is playing a role in a play that he never auditioned for. The woman has decided—without telling him, and perhaps without admitting it to herself—who she needed him to be for her. Either she wants him to be really tough and imagines him this way, and she doesn't give him the space to not be tough; or, maybe she does the reverse, and clips him, makes him inoffensive: the safe guy who will never hurt her, never leave, never cheat—like a sweet puppy. Then she says: *I'm not interested.*

What's behind the disconnect?

Men don't explain to women that their sexuality is driven by their internal states: If a man feels anxious or depressed, if he is struggling with his self-worth—his sexuality will change. The fear of rejection and inadequacy, the need to feel competent, to know that she's enjoying him and into it—these are all important and intensely relational qualities of a man's sexuality.

People tend to think of female sexuality as being very complicated, while oversimplifying male sexuality. There's the assumption that women want to connect and men want to get laid—the idea that women have the monopoly on intimacy and best understand closeness. These are highly gendered stereotypes that really don't serve anybody, but they are quite tenacious.

While there are differences between men and women, I think we all fall prey to very old stereotypes and evolutionary ideas that support certain stereotypes even though they're not necessarily that accurate: Women are told that there is one form of expression for sadness and hurt, and that in the masculine discourse, it's more acceptable to be angry and to pretend self-sufficiency. We often mistake this kind of difference as essential and innate, when in fact it is much more cultural. Then we come up with all kinds of evolutionary and biological theories to support the stereotype.

What about men projecting onto women?

Oh, yes—it's equal opportunity. We're more familiar with the projections of men on women than we are with the projections of women on men. For instance:

If a man sees a woman as brittle, he may love her with a sense of extra burden—he must take care of her. He takes on a parental role. This is one trap, or way, that relationships become parental, and it can happen with any gender.

There are long histories of men desexualizing women (think the

Madonna complex) and putting them into a mother role. Or, on the flip side, men may assume a woman who is very sexual is someone who won't stay with him, because his sense of self-worth is put into question: *Am I enough?* Everybody plays these games: If I'm not enough, if I criticize or berate you a little bit, then I become more.

How do you mend the disconnect? Is it just a matter of starting the conversation?

Yes, but it has to be a particular kind of conversation. I think this topic is fraught. In the United States, sexuality is looked at through a moral, puritanical lens—America is at war with the concept of pleasure in general. Everything is about control. But sexuality in many ways is a negotiation with your surrendering—it's about a loss of control.

The conversation is less about what to do and how to fix it. First, it needs to be about changing the landscape and the way we perceive things. What are the conversations women are allowed to have, and what are the conversations men are allowed to have?

Right now, for example, men are allowed to lie by exaggerating and by bragging, and women are allowed to emphasize self-denial and minimizing. That's the basic rule around sexuality: Women lie down, and men lie up. The day you go into a men's locker room and you hear them talking about how their wives are jumping them and they're not interested . . . that will be evolution.

Do you find that the same-sex couples you see have similar and/or different problems than the hetero couples?

When I work with same-sex couples, which is about a third of my practice, it helps me to see what is generally relational, what is role-based, what is more gender-specific, and what is more gender-specific in a heterosexual context. On some level, I would say, yes, of course men have to deal with men issues; and from a cultural perspective, when you put two men in the room, that's double the amount of men issues you're dealing with. Same for women. But many of the questions and issues that come up in relationships are not necessarily more feminine or masculine, and these questions and issues are similar for same-sex and heterosexual partners. Often I see the same dynamics regardless: a pursuer and a distancer (a person who wants more and a person who is withholding) or a magnifier (who escalates) and a minimizer (who shuts down). Fight, flight, freeze—there is no gender attached to this pattern.

Beyond gender, though, a lot of our relationship behavior and dynamics stem from our family history and upbringing. Our emotional history is inscribed in the physicality of our sexuality. Tell me how you were loved, and I will tell you how you make love.

FROM THE GOOPASUTRA
THE LIST

New York therapist Eric G. Schneider (board-certified sex-ologist, MEd, DMin, PhD candidate in human sexuality) has a fantastic technique for getting more of what you want sexually—and understanding what your partner wants—in a fun, relatively low-drama, almost Mad-Libs way. Here's how he describes The List:

"Sometimes talking about sex is tough, so try writing about it! It's all about creating space, and contributing to that space, that makes sexual exploration safe and fun.

"Divide a paper into four columns with the headings 'I Love'; 'I Like'; 'I Would Try'; and 'I Would Never Try.' Both you and your partner can spend some time apart, creating your lists. Then plan an exchange. No judgments, no criticism, all done in the spirit of sharing and openness. Keep in mind that lists of sexual preferences are often conditioned behaviorally over time, and they often shift.

"Next, check for overlaps—and focus on those. Don't worry about the ones that don't overlap. And on another piece of paper, note the overlaps: 'We both love...'; 'We both like...'; 'We both would like to try...'; 'We would never try...'"

GOOP note: We have also tried adapting/game-ifying this technique by two partners creating a single list. One person (you, since you're suggesting it) goes first. Write: "I really like...," and fill in the blank. Your partner goes next. Keep adding to the list as long as you both can, taking turns each time. You can alter the fill-in-the-blank to "...turns me on"; "I'd like to try...," etc.

CHAPTER 4

deepening intimacy

One of the foremost thinkers on matters of sex, psychotherapist and sexuality counselor Ian Kerner (author of *She Comes First*), has a layered understanding of intimacy as both risk and reward. Kerner says intimacy requires that you feel secure enough in someone's presence to be vulnerable, but that intimacy is not equivalent to closeness or familiarity. Actually, it's the opposite in some ways: Kerner notes that many relationships begin on an intimacy high, when curiosity is strong and partners are revealing and discovering new things about each other, but then it can start to burn out as there's less to find out. Here, he explains how to get around this intimacy barrier, as well as other roadblocks.

The Risk and Reward of Intimacy

IAN KERNER, PHD

How do you define sexual intimacy? Why is it important?

Intimacy is generally defined as a sense of closeness or familiarity with another person, and so sexual intimacy would be the experience of that sense of closeness through sexual connection. I think of intimacy somewhat differently, though, as I believe that you can be close to someone or familiar with someone without necessarily feeling intimacy. To me, intimacy is feeling safe enough and secure enough in a person's presence to be able to reveal and express vulnerability. In this sense, intimacy requires a bit of risk—and is also the reward.

Sexual intimacy can be sharing a fantasy with a partner for the first time, or initiating sex when you're not sure how your partner will respond, or deciding not to fake an orgasm and instead letting your partner know what works or doesn't. Sexual intimacy might be feeling safe enough to share a sexual problem you're having. Sexual intimacy is about being authentic and having that authenticity mirrored back to you. While sexual arousal has physical/chemical indicators, I'm not sure intimacy does; the experience of intimacy is subjective.

Can you have intimacy without attachment?

Yes. Two people can meet and make love and feel intimacy without necessarily having a deep attachment. Attachments are generally developed, cultivated, and reinforced over time. You might be attached to someone without experiencing intimacy, but a strong, secure attachment will provide the foundation for the expression of intimacy. When it comes to sex, we tend to think of attachment as occurring between two people, but studies of people in consensually nonmonogamous relationships show that intimacy is additive, not finite. Humans are incredibly flexible and elastic, but most of us pursue intimacy within the structure of sexual exclusivity.

Is intimacy different for men and women?

I don't think intimacy is gendered. Intimacy is a feeling created through connection between people. The cliché is that women are naturally more tuned in to intimacy and men are more tone-deaf, but I haven't found this to be the case.

If you're guarded or defensive, you're not going to be able to experience intimacy. Men and women may express their defenses in different ways—men may be more likely to lash out, while women may be more likely to self-silence (although this is a generalization); but once defenses are down, and we feel safe and secure, and we can be vulnerable, men and women are much more similar than different.

The cliché is that women are naturally more tuned in to intimacy and men are more tone-deaf, but I haven't found this to be the case.

What are the typical roadblocks to intimacy? And what degrades intimacy once it's established?

Intimacy requires vulnerability—and knowing that you're safe to be vulnerable. It is possible to have sex without experiencing intimacy. Many often do. Many couples are not in the sort of relationship that supports the experience of sexual intimacy. If you're anxious about sex, you're not going to be able to experience intimacy. If you're watching yourself having sex and you're thinking about your sexual performance, then you're not going to experience intimacy. If you're angry at your partner or feel that your partner doesn't understand you or care to understand you, then you're not going to be able to experience intimacy. Anxiety. Anger. Stress. Resentment. Indifference. Boredom. Those are all roadblocks to intimacy.

In a study I conducted with Kristen Mark, PhD, from the University of Kentucky, nearly 70 percent of those surveyed expressed being bored in their relationships. But nearly 90 percent said they would be interested if their partner made a sexy suggestion. For couples who have somehow found they've taken a turn off the intimacy highway, making that sexy suggestion is a way of getting back on.

How do you deepen intimacy?

Relationships often begin with a profound burst of intimacy in the form of mutual self-expansion. There's so much we don't know about the other person and so much we want to learn, and our mutual curiosity and desire to know and be known creates intimacy. We are constantly discovering and revealing. As relationships grow familiar, the journey of mutual self-expansion slows down. Closeness plus familiarity does not equal intimacy. Intimacy requires having more to reveal, more to discover. Deepening intimacy requires finding ways to continue the journey of mutual self-expansion. In sexual terms, this could mean exploring a new erotic theme together, or being able to discuss a sexual issue together.

FROM THE GOOPASUTRA
QUIRKY PLACES TO GET IT ON

Sometimes, a change of scenery can do wonders. Here are a dozen-plus places we've had sex that rank high in staffers' memories:

1. My favorite salumeria in Italy.
2. Beach sex—kind of hard to execute but so worth it.
3. A unisex bathroom at a wedding. It was interesting until people started knocking.
4. On a children's pirate ship.

5. A couch: I'm very vanilla.

6. A (parked) speedboat.

7. His office floor.

8. A rain forest: It was exhilarating. We were right next to a river, so afterward we went for a naked dip.

9. College, in the upper rows of a massive auditorium after Psych 101 (not with the professor). I also used to do it with my high school boyfriend in the weight training room. Fetish?

10. My backyard.

11. An outdoor shower, while our guests were on the nearby back deck...

12. On a hike by the ocean. We found a quiet spot and proceeded to have very hot, memorable sex. The risk of being seen definitely heightened it.

13. In the library stacks (it was nighttime, and it was on a high floor, in an esoteric subject area).

14. In a car.

15. In sleeping bags, at the Great Wall of China!

CHAPTER 5

aphrodisiacs to get your freak on

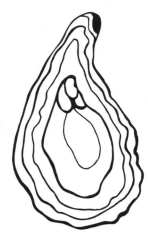

There's some science behind the buzz/old wives' tales about aphrodisiac foods like chocolate and oysters, and there actually are many foods and supplements that support sex drive and increased libido, says London nutritionist Adam Cunliffe, who has spent most of his career in the research space (though he does see a few lucky clients).

"Aphrodisiacs make their impact using a range of mechanisms affecting the brain, blood flow, and hormones," Cunliffe explains, while some "actually enhance both male and female fertility and improve the chances of successful conception." How strong are they? "Like most natural remedies, the impact of natural aphrodisiacs tends to be subtler than pharmaceutical drugs like Viagra, but real nevertheless." Cunliffe says that with an aphrodisiac, you should be able to experience the results the same day.

One surprise that shouldn't have been so surprising: Adaptogens like ashwagandha—and really anything that reduces stress—often have results between the sheets. Cunliffe breaks down some of the most powerful aphrodisiacs:

10 Aphrodisiacs for Better Sex

ADAM CUNLIFFE, PHD, RNUTR

Adaptogens

1. **Ashwagandha:** This Ayurvedic herb has been clinically shown to improve the quantity and health of sperm, but it's also powerful for reducing stress, which can be at the root of all kinds of fertility and conception problems. Ashwagandha is potent, so I recommend taking it only as needed, particularly because it's slightly relaxing and can begin to lose its efficacy if you take it all the time. (Note: Ashwagandha should not be taken during any phase of pregnancy, as its safety for pregnant women has not been established.)

2. **Mucuna Pruriens:** Also called velvet bean (or cowitch, because touching the bean as it's growing in its natural form can trigger a dermatitis reaction), this is a legume of African and Asian origin. It contains L-dopa, which is converted to dopamine, the reward chemical in the brain—it's the same system that ecstasy would work on, and while it's certainly more mild, it has the effect of boosting that system. Many people find that Mucuna pruriens puts them in "the mood for love," but it can also be an energy booster. Try taking with a passiflora (passionflower) tea, which enhances the effect. The Mucuna pruriens bean itself is not really edible, so you'll take it ground up in some kind of capsule.

3. **Maca:** Cultivated in South America for more than three thousand years, maca helps improve sexual function in both men and women, and also promotes healthy ovulation in women. It typically comes in a powder, made by grinding up the dried root. Scientists studying maca found that while it increased sexual drive and performance, there was no effect on sex hormones—when they started looking in more detail, they realized it was impacting the psychology of sex, including helping people create effective sexual fantasies. Some people don't like the taste—it's rich, malty, with a slight bitterness—so it's best mixed into smoothies or other foods (although I personally quite like the flavor). It's safe enough to take every day—you'll find a portion of it in Moon Juice's Sex Dust.

Supplements

4. **Horny Goat Weed:** Considered to be an old faithful among herbal aphrodisiacs, it was reputedly given its name by Chinese goat herders who noticed that their flocks' sexual behavior increased when grazing in fields of it. Horny goat weed contains a compound called icariin, which has been shown to have Viagra-like activity and can promote stronger, longer-lasting erections. Icariin is a PDE inhibitor—meaning, in men, it keeps the blood flowing more effectively in the right place by opening up the blood vessels (just be careful to stop taking it before a surgery, as it keeps blood flow thin). Horny goat weed is found in most mixed herbal aphrodisiacs; often, you'll find it in a capsule mixed with other potent herbs, like maca (as it is in the Moon Juice brand's Sex Dust).

5. **Histidine:** The opposite of the groggy, tired effect of taking an antihistamine, the amino acid histidine has generally stimulating effects, making you more aware and sensitive (it can be good for people looking to lose weight). Histidine is an essential amino acid for children, but as adults we can synthesize it in our bodies,

so it becomes nonessential. Taken as a supplement, it has been shown to enhance orgasm, and histidine also has been reported to facilitate orgasms in women who've never had one before, since it stimulates the vulva reflex. (People with allergies, eczema, asthma, or food intolerances should be careful, as histidine can aggravate those conditions.)

6. **Pycnogenol:** This supplement is extracted from the bark of French maritime pine trees, and it's both an effective natural aphrodisiac and a fertility enhancer in men and women. Pycnogenol is clinically proven to treat erectile dysfunction and enhance sperm motility (aka their ability to swim fast and strong enough to reach the egg), and it has been shown to have strong aphrodisiac qualities in women. It's especially effective when combined with arginine, an amino acid that's primarily used for heart health.

Foods

7. **Pomegranates:** Cut or bite into a pomegranate, and you'll find that it's obviously sexy! Reputed since antiquity to be a "food of love," the pomegranate is high in antioxidants and has more recently been shown to increase testosterone and sex drive in both men and women. Eat it fresh with the seeds, or drink it as a juice.

8. **Chocolate:** Any gift might cause a release of oxytocin in the recipient, which leads to feelings of attraction and bonding, but chocolate also has a chemical composition with feel-good compounds. Theobromine, a central nervous system stimulant, is similar to caffeine but is said to have mood-boosting capabilities as well. Chocolate contains phenethylamine, too, which, along with theobromine, can trigger endorphin and dopamine release.

9. **Oysters:** Though many dismiss it as an old wives' tale, the high concentration of zinc in oysters is actually associated with

fertility and sperm production, particularly in men. Oysters also contain essential amino acids that promote good sexual function.

10. **Sultan's Paste (Mesir Macunu):** Once a Turkish secret (though it's now more widely available), Sultan's Paste is made up of more than forty herbs and spices, including fenugreek, saffron, and ginger, that can help to improve blood flow and increase energy and desire. While it's hard to pin down exactly which are the most active ingredients, fenugreek in particular has measurable aphrodisiac qualities for men and women. Sultan's Paste has a molasses-like consistency, and it comes in a jar. You can eat it straight off the spoon (it has a sweet, spicy, exotic taste), spread it on toast, or mix it with water for a tonic. It's great as a pick-me-up.

FROM THE GOOPASUTRA
Sex Bark

Amanda Chantal Bacon—founder of the LA-based holistic lifestyle Moon Juice shops—shared this quick, potent chocolate recipe with us. Complete with Moon Juice's Sex Dust (the aphrodisiac warming potion referenced by nutritionist Adam Cunliffe), it remains a favorite for a sweet bite after a romantic dinner.

SERVES 4–6

¼ cup coconut oil
¼ cup ghee
1 cup Moon Pantry cacao
3 teaspoons Moon Pantry Sex Dust
2 teaspoons Moon Pantry ashwagandha
¼ cup raw honey or several drops stevia
1½ tablespoons Moon Pantry cacao nibs

Combine coconut oil and ghee in a glass bowl set over a simmering pot of water, and stir until completely melted. Remove from the heat and whisk in cacao, powders, and the sweetener of your choice. We like this very chocolaty and not too sweet, but feel free to adjust with more stevia or honey. Pour into an 8 x 8 glass or metal baking dish, sprinkle with cacao nibs, and freeze for about 20 minutes, or until firm. When ready, pop the bark out of the dish with a butter knife, and break into pieces. (If you want to play around with the thickness of the bark, pour it into different-sized baking dishes to set.)

CHAPTER 6

navigating the mind-fuck of dating

When you're on a roll, dating at any age can be wildly exciting. If you're stuck, or not finding what you're looking for, dating can be a mind-fuck (also at any age). As in any office, we've collectively been on our share of good and horrid dates. (One particularly bad dating story began with a staffer going on what they thought was a rekindling of a long-term relationship, which quickly dissolved into a breakup, and ended with their being "sent home" in an UberPool.) Our go-to relationship expert and life adviser, Suzannah Galland, outlines the path to more fun dates, less bad ones, and something more (if that's what you're after).

A Better Way to Play the Dating Game

SUZANNAH GALLAND

How do you recommend approaching dating if you're not looking for something serious?

Take a long, deep breath and imagine a date without expectations and with no time frame. Picture yourself having fun and your desires being satisfied. This is the mental place you should go to whenever you're considering a potential date, looking for one, or getting ready for a night out.

Give yourself permission to enjoy the position you are in, far from any relationship hype, and to sit back with confidence and enjoy dating and the oncoming pursuits.

Is there a gut check for when you are looking for a more committed partner?

Ask yourself this simple question: *What do I want from a partner?* Write it down. Take a good look at the characteristics of a potential partner—do they align with what you wrote down?

Another approach is to think about what values align with your core (e.g., loyalty, meaning, stimulus, success, safety). This will prevent you from wasting time and analyzing whats and whys that are not relevant to you. The next time you're ready to give love, do a check of your potential partner's values—which could be a combination of what is listed on an online dating profile, what they articulate as important to them, how they actually live, and so on. Do their values match up with yours?

When does dating become something more—how do you know?

When something fabulous happens to you, you no longer want to call your best friend or your mother. Instead, you want to share it with your

Unlike lust, there's a synchronicity about love— you think of the person and they call.

new partner first. That's your barometer— the point where "I" tends to become "we."

Also, when in love, we feel confident, validated, and desired. Unlike lust, there's a synchronicity about love—you think of the person and they call.

Love is feeling the flow—when you do, that's when you know there's something special happening.

What's the most common fear you see around dating?

I see a lot of clients who are dealing with the pain of a breakup. People come to me when a lover they thought to be "the one" has failed them in some way, and they freeze—afraid to love again. I gently remind them that there are other lovers for the soul out there, but at this point, I really encourage personal healing. The work of getting out of this sort of despair trap and recovering from a painful breakup entails clearing and cleaning up after—and, often, adopting a forgiving attitude toward yourself.

What are some of your long-standing relationship tips?

- Trying to improve your love life can be akin to home improvement in some ways. The bedroom is generally a reflection of the most intimate part of you—it's where you sleep, dream, desire, long, touch. If you need a kick start, look at the space around you: Is it inviting? Sensual? Even just tidying up your space or upgrading your bed linens can create a shift.
- On a similar note, if you're trying to move beyond a former lover to a new one, I recommend getting rid of your old underwear/ lingerie. The lingerie you wore with past lovers can carry the toxic residue of those relationships, along with painful memories.
- A sense of personal mystery will go a long way toward helping you tap into your own desire, which emanates outward, making

you all the more attractive to others. Let's use lingerie as an example—if you're into it, buy an over-the-top-sexy pair of panties to wear on a date (when you're not planning on taking your clothes off). Let it be a "secret" you think of throughout the date.

- Knowing how to "pitch yourself" is essential to getting what you want—I think of it as emotional branding. Be able to share who you are in one minute on a date. Pick one thing that's important to you, for example, and put it at the top of your dating profile. If one of your pet peeves is men exaggerating their accomplishments, state that you want a relationship defined by authenticity and confidence.

- It's important to know that our thoughts project an energetic wave that travels much like light and sound. We can direct how and what we think toward anyone, and this is one way we manifest our passion. Don't underestimate the power of a loving thought—which has a way of circling back to you.

FROM THE GOOPASUTRA
THE MAKING OF A SEXY BEDROOM

Top LA interior designer Schuyler Samperton has easy tips for making anyone's bedroom more seductive. "The room should connect with all the senses, ideally," she says. "Soft, pleasing texture to touch, lovely scents through fresh flowers or candles, great music, a spot for drinks or a few treats, and of course, a beautiful look." Here are her seven bedroom ideas to live by:

1. For the bed, think inviting and romantic: A four-poster or upholstered bed is very sexy. Curtain panels always lend a lush, languid Merchant Ivory feel. The bed should look pulled together but not overdone. And too many throw pillows are a total buzzkill.

2. For linens, rumpled is best! Anything too fussy or maintenance-heavy can be off-putting and a spontaneity killer. I prefer simple white sheets, in linen or cotton (no satin).

3. A great music source is an absolute must.

4. Flattering lighting is critical in this particular context. That means dimmable, ambient fixtures—never overhead! Ambient light is always more beautiful. Of course, several well-placed, mildly scented candles can't hurt. Just avoid overdoing it—you don't want to re-create a 1980s Whitesnake video moment.

5. Eliminate all overflowing wastebaskets, clutter, and photos of your parents and/or yourself circa eighth grade.

6. It's nice to have a pretty side table nearby for a drink or two.

7. No stuffed animals.

to (sex) toy or not?

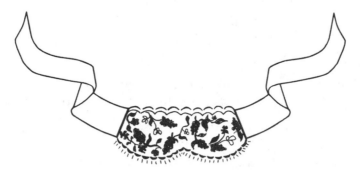

W e've learned a lot about sex toys since we included the infamous 24-karat gold dildo in a gift guide a few years back... While some sex experts are bigger proponents of toys for enhancing self-pleasure and spicing up partner sex than others, who stand by a less-bells-and-whistles approach, it's fair to say it's a myth that women are becoming addicted to vibrators. If you're toy-curious, sexuality coach Layla Martin outlines a nonintimidating way to experiment. Martin, who has studied Tantric and Taoist traditions, works with people (primarily online, which she finds is more comfortable for many) regarding the use of practical tools that strengthen their sexuality—so the toys she recommends are intended to actually enhance a person's sexual presence and overall seduction appeal—as opposed to serving as a distraction.

Bringing Toys into the Bedroom

LAYLA MARTIN

What are the pros and cons of using toys?

In solo play, sex toys bring variation and variety to the types of plea-sure you experience, which is fabulous. With a toy, you can be inspired to try something different—anal exploration, light bondage, or a new kind of orgasm. Orgasms are healthy, wonderful experiences, and some women are able to orgasm much more easily with a vibrator.

Toys also inspire a different type of self-pleasure. I encourage my clients to use a glass or stone dildo to open up and sensitize the cervix, which makes it easier for them to have cervical orgasms. I also love the use of a jade egg, which turns self-pleasuring into a deeper sexual adventure—meaning you can start to work with sexual energy and sacred or spiritual states through your self-pleasuring.

One thing I find most people never consider is that every time you self-pleasure or orgasm, you are training your body and mind to orgasm in that one specific way. Therefore, while toys can be a lot of fun, you want to mix up how you self-pleasure so your body doesn't become accus-tomed to a sole type of stimulation. It's not that you get addicted—women aren't addicted to vibrators—but they train their body to orgasm from the specific stimulation of the vibra-tor, and that can make it harder to orgasm in other ways.

> *It's not that you get addicted—women aren't addicted to vibrators—but they train their body to orgasm from the specific stimulation of the vibrator, and that can make it harder to orgasm in other ways.*

Each time you orgasm or experience sexual pleasure, you are strengthening the neuronal pathways for that type of stimulation. The brain likes what is easy, so if you travel the same path again and again, the tendency to orgasm in that one specific way is reinforced.

If you use a sex toy that is very different from sex with a partner, you can make your brain want to experience orgasm or pleasure in a way that is out of sync with what your partner can offer. Alternatively, I have female clients who have penetrative sex with their partners and use dildos during self-pleasure: If you self-pleasure regularly with a dildo, you train your body to experience pleasure through penetration and to experience orgasm through penetration—and this makes it easier to have orgasms during penetrative sex.

For the uninitiated, how do you get comfortable with the idea of using a toy?

It can be scary to try a toy for the first time! I find that knowing how to use it makes a big difference—so purchasing from a store that has helpful information or doing some research will help you feel excited rather than apprehensive. You might also want to check out the website OMGYes.com, where loads of women discuss how they like to touch themselves, which may be inspiring and reduce fear. Also...focus on the pleasure of it! That will excite you.

How do you get a partner comfortable with using a toy?

Explain to your partner that you want to enhance your sexual experience. You aren't trying to replace them or use a toy because they aren't fulfilling you. It's an exploration and a shared experience. Maybe share that you would love for them to try it on you—and be specific about what you would like to experience. A lot of men, especially, want to know exactly how to please a woman, and specific, direct instructions are very helpful so they feel like they know what they are doing. Express that it is about your partner doing something with you or to you, rather than about your wanting the experience of the toy—that way they don't feel threatened, but instead as though they are experiencing it with you.

Which toys do you recommend?

As more of a holistic sex expert, I recommend toys that encourage sexual presence, open up the body, and increase sensitivity and a connection to sexual energy—rather than toys that overwhelm the system.

In my toy box, I have:

- A jade egg, which I use for self-pleasuring and a yoga practice for my pussy.
- A Laid D.1 moonstone dildo, which is great for opening me up to cervical orgasms and deep vaginal pleasure.
- Anal plugs are fabulous for experiencing anal pleasure and orgasms.
- I like smaller glass dildos for doing de-armoring, which is basically a sexual practice where you press the dildo into pressure points inside the vagina and create deep inner relaxation. This helps to release stored trauma and emotional baggage from the vagina and opens you up to much more epic sexual experiences. It's like doing a physical vaginal cleanse for yourself.
- Blindfolds for encouraging deeper sensitivity and surrender.
- I like something that will cause intensity—like a little whip if you enjoy light pain, or a riding crop if you like it really painful.
- I also love skin activators like fake furs and feathers that can be used to awaken the sensitivity of the skin.

What's the ideal environment for incorporating a toy?

You generally want lube or skin-friendly oil to use with a toy. And if you are at it . . . why not get a blindfold to enhance your sensations and something soft to lie on so you are fully switched on for the experience?

Are there toy materials you steer clear of?

Lots of toys are manufactured with toxic chemicals and dyes that are known carcinogens and hormone disrupters. Steer clear of cheaply manufactured sex toys made of plastic (or unlabeled materials). There is absolutely no regulation of the sex toy industry, and manufacturers can literally put anything into a sex toy, even if it's been regulated as a health hazard in other areas.

Silicone is safe if it is pure silicone and not mixed with other chemicals. Since you have no way of knowing this, you'll want to purchase from a seller that pays attention to this sort of thing, like Babeland or She Bop.

Other materials that are safe include glass, metal, and ceramic (with lead-free glaze). Certain stones are safe if they are manufactured correctly, such as Norwegian moonstone and jade. However, many stones are not safe for internal use and may not be manufactured correctly, so again, you have to be careful about where you buy. Jimmyjane, Icicles, NobEssence, Laid, and Earth Erotics all make healthy sex toys; and Babeland, mentioned above, has good information and sourcing practices with their products.

FROM THE GOOPASUTRA
SHAVING VS. WAXING VS. NOT

There are no shoulds at all when it comes to intimate body hair; what turns on one person repels another—from total denuded Brazilian to full-'70s bush—so you've got to go with what you think is sexy/cool-looking/feels right. Below are some ungendered pros and cons (beyond the visual, because, again, each of these looks/techniques is hot to someone and not-hot to someone else):

Shaving: Shaving does the job easily for legs, underarms, or even a straightforward bikini line, but it's less simple for serious nooks and crannies: Razor burn, razor bumps, and God forbid, nicks are an absolute bummer in any sort of intimate area. If you're super adept with a razor and feel comfortable, by all means go for it, but if you're thinking of trying, say, a full-on Brazilian, wax might be a better option. The other unpleasant factor is that hair cut by a razor has a sharper edge than natural hair—or hair that's been waxed or even lasered—so it's more likely not only to be uncomfortable as it grows back, but also to cause ingrown hairs. Then again, it's cheap, straightforward, and private.

Waxing: A not-permanent, effective way to get a lot of hair off at once, waxing hurts like hell. But if you're wanting a no-hair, or very minimal hair–landing-strip situation, waxing is probably your best bet. There are cold waxes, sugar waxes, green-algae waxes—all of them with fans who say they don't hurt. Assume that no matter the form, a wax *is* going to hurt, and brace yourself (mentally, or with anything from arnica to a cocktail).

Waxing results last significantly longer than shaving (all depend on how fast an individual's hair grows back), and it grows back in softer and, eventually, thinner, theoretically causing fewer ingrowns; but again, waxing can cause irritation in and of itself.

Laser Hair Removal: If you're really, adamantly super sure you want to get rid of hair in a particular spot, laser hair removal is markedly less painful than waxing—and you typically have to do it only six or so times, with perhaps a once-a-year touch-up after that, depending on your body. (The up-front cost of laser removal is obviously higher, but depending on how regularly you get waxed, the laser route could shake out to less money in the long run.)

That said, really be sure: Women who opted to go completely bare when it was all the rage might be experiencing some regret during the more-natural phase happening now; and, trends aside, more than a few ob-gyns we've talked to say some of the current vagina-dysmorphia–powered plastic surgery customers are women who've lasered all of their hair away permanently, and then ended up not liking what they saw.

You can do laser hair removal in a salon—expensive but about a thousand times easier. Or at home, which is as effective but harder to do, depending on the spots you're targeting, blissfully private, and much cheaper. Laser hair removal used to work on only pale-skinned people with dark hair, but technology has caught up at last, and it now works on all skin and hair colors.

CHAPTER 8

friends with benefits—is it a benefit?

While the phenomenon of friends with benefits tends to be romanticized in popular culture—the besties who seduce each other one random night, fall in love, and live happily ever after—the outcomes in reality seem to mixed. In a GOOP office poll, we were pretty evenly split among:

- People who said they'd never entertain the idea—"Nope."
- Those who had good experiences being a friend with benefits— "We had a tight friendship to begin with, which admittedly I was afraid of jeopardizing, but our sexual tension and curiosity was undeniable. If you are capable of compartmentalizing and appreciating each experience for what it is without labeling and developing a story behind it—you can have your cake and eat it, too."

- Those who said it ended badly for them, mostly due to someone in the relationship "catching feelings"—"Even if I knew I didn't like him like that and never would, it was hard for me to shake my growing attachment. Ironically, if the guy was the one growing attached to me, I would panic and get out ASAP."

Social psychologist Justin Lehmiller, author of *Tell Me What You Want: The Science of Sexual Desire and How It Can Help You Improve Your Sex Life*, and faculty affiliate of the Kinsey Institute, researches and writes about casual sex on his blog *Sex & Psychology*. He says that how you view sex and love—are they separate or do they go together?—helps predict how you'd fare in a friends-with-benefits situation. According to Lehmiller, the other two important predictors for how the relationship turns out are expectations (not a good sign when the friends are actually looking for romantic partnership) and communication (ground rules are key). If you're considering whether to act on your attraction to a friend, or how you'd receive a come-on from a currently platonic someone, read on. And for more from Lehmiller on the art of unconventional sex, see his Q&A's on open relationships and threesomes on pages 95 and 149.

How to Have Sex with Your Friend Without Ruining Everything

JUSTIN LEHMILLER, PHD

What are the options when it comes to friends-with-benefits situations?

Friends with benefits relationships aren't as simple and straightforward as the name implies. They vary a lot when it comes to the relationship history and intimate connection that exist between partners. What's most common is for people who first have a solid friendship to add a sexual component. However, others don't have much of a friendship—they might give each other "booty calls" from time to time but not really have any relationship beyond that. Then there are those who become friends with benefits following a breakup or divorce, aka they're having "ex-sex."

How long do they typically last?

While some friends-with-benefits relationships last only a few weeks or months, others last years. Based on a longitudinal study I conducted, these relationships tend to be relatively short-lived, though, with the vast majority ending or transitioning into another kind of relationship within one year. (Only about one in four were still friends with benefits at the end of our study.)

Are there any predictors of how a friends-with-benefits relationship will turn out?

That same study also revealed two things that really matter when it comes to achieving a positive outcome, which I would define as maintaining some type of long-term relationship with your partner as opposed to losing all contact with them. First, expectations matter: People who said they wanted to maintain their friendship or remain friends with benefits in the long run tended to be pretty successful in achieving those goals. When people said they eventually wanted to become romantic partners, things didn't work out so well. Only about 1 in 7 of the participants who wanted to make the leap to romance were able to do so after a year.

Second, communication and ground rules are extremely important. We found that the more time people spent setting up ground rules initially, the more likely they were to maintain a relationship with their partner over time; the less people did this, the more likely they were to report being estranged in the end.

Can you avoid catching feelings, and what should you do if you start to feel something more?

Some people are more prone to "catching feelings" than others. It really depends on whether you're the kind of person who views sex and love as going together (something psychologists call a restricted sociosexual orientation) or as things that are separate (known as an unrestricted sociosexual orientation). If you're the former type, odds are that you'll end up wanting more than just friendship in the end; if you're the latter type, not so much.

> *Some people are more prone to "catching feelings" than others.*

If you end up desiring a romantic relationship at some point, it's probably best to be open about that with your partner sooner rather than later. Of course, there's a chance they might want the same thing, too—and, if so, you can transition into another kind of relationship that makes everyone happy. If they don't want to move to a romance, though, then it might be time to call it quits before things get really messy.

What's the best exit strategy? Is it usually possible to go back to being just friends?

We don't really have data yet on the best way to wind down a friends-with-benefits situation. One strategy that might be helpful is to set an expiration or renewal date for the benefits at the start. This way, you have a natural opportunity to revisit things after a certain amount of time and mutually decide whether you'd like to keep going or go back to being just friends. It's definitely possible to go back to a basic friendship—studies show that many people have done it. Again, though, the odds of this happening depend in large part on how much care and effort you put into setting the ground rules up front.

When is being friends with benefits a bad idea?

If you're looking at a friends-with-benefits situation as a way to land a romantic partner, think again: The data suggest that, while possible, this is an unlikely outcome. If true love is what you're after, you're probably better off with traditional dating, rather than trying to lure someone into a relationship by claiming you want "no strings" sex when there are actually a lot of strings attached.

Also, given that friends-with-benefits arrangements tend to be nonmonogamous, people who are prone to jealousy and insecurity are probably going to have a harder time navigating these relationships.

What doesn't really matter, though, is age. People at any age can have friends with benefits. In fact, in the studies I've conducted on this topic, I've routinely had people in their fifties and sixties and beyond in my samples, which tells us these relationships aren't just for college students.

Are there other common motivations behind friends-with-benefits situations one should be aware of?

Many friends with benefits get together only when they've been drinking. The potential problem here is that when people are drunk, their communication abilities are impaired and they don't always make the best relationship decisions. What this means is that if you're mixing alcohol and sex with a friend, there's the potential for things to get really complicated.

Also, my research shows that there are gender differences in what men and women want from friends-with-benefits relationships. Specifically, men are more likely than women to say they're in it for the sex and they want to stay friends with benefits indefinitely; by contrast, women are more likely than men to say they are in it to emotionally connect with another person and they want the arrangement to be temporary, ultimately transitioning back to "just friends," or becoming romantic. These gender differences in motivations and expectations may help to explain why so many friends-with-benefits relationships just don't work out in the end. They also further highlight the importance of getting on the same page up front.

CHAPTER 9

reigniting attraction

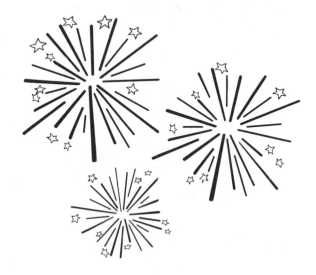

No one expects the honeymoon phase to last forever, and yet when the once-thrilling spark dims in a relationship, it can feel devastating. Or, as one GOOP staffer put it: "I'm married, and I find myself having little crushes here and there and I always feel so guilty about it. I tell myself that I'm human and everyone gets crushes from time to time. I would never act on them, but I just want to know I'm not alone in that issue."

Waning attraction, disinterest, sex droughts—none of it is fun, and it leaves us wondering: *There has to be a better way, right?* Enter no-nonsense psychotherapist Barry Michels (cowriter, with Phil Stutz, of *The Tools* and *Coming Alive*), who has a penchant for helping people get unstuck. Michels shares how to restart sexual intimacy after you've lost it and the one turn-on he's found that is guaranteed to work—forever.

Waning Sexual Attraction and the One Enduring Turn-On

BARRY MICHELS

Why does sexual attraction always seem to wane in a long-term relationship?

When people come to me and tell me they're no longer attracted to their partners, the reasons they give are almost never the real ones. Typically, female clients attribute their loss of interest to their partners' physical habits (the smacking sound they make when chewing food, the way they dress, bad breath, how they leave their socks on the floor, etc.). Men more often attribute it to feeling like their partner is too demanding, nags or criticizes them too much, or needs to discuss everything to death. I'm not saying these complaints are necessarily irrelevant, but they rarely reveal the full picture. If you think back to the beginning of your relationship, you were likely aware of most of these traits, but at the time, you found them part of an adorable package.

So what's really going on?

The reality that most people don't like to face is that sexual attraction wanes in almost every long-term relationship. When people meet each other for the first time, they experience a rush of desire. They're in the "idealization" phase of their relationship, where each feels they've found "the one"—a partner who's perfect for them. Each person is putting his or her best foot forward, careful not to repeat the mistakes they've made in past relationships. Their sex life works seamlessly, without effort. And deep down, each thinks this state of bliss is going to last forever.

Somewhere after six to nine months, the rose-colored glasses usually come off and the couple move into the disillusionment phase.

Because each partner feels comfortable, they begin to reveal their true selves. Originally, they couldn't get enough of each other; now, maybe even the smallest things can be irritating. The passion begins to wane. Sometimes they begin to criticize each other, but even if the criticisms aren't voiced—each feels the other silently judging them. A distance is created. Add the increased stress of, say, work, children, and/or aging parents, and you end up with a relationship where true intimacy is a bygone memory.

But it isn't this distance that destroys sexual intimacy; it's something even more painful. To understand it, you have to think about what sex really is. Our society tends to treat sex as if it were merely a physical act, devoid of any vulnerable emotions. That might be accurate for a casual hookup, but once you develop deeper feelings for a person, you're in an entirely different realm. Sex, within the context of a committed relationship, renders you extremely vulnerable. Your partner sees *everything* about you that you've carefully hidden from the world: the real you, trembling with ecstasy, crying out with passion, possessed by and acting out of pure animal desire. The face your partner sees is not one you reveal to everyone—and it renders you nakedly vulnerable to him or her.

Once there's distance in a relationship, that kind of vulnerability no longer feels safe. So people retreat to a less revealing (and therefore less passionate) version of sex, which quickly becomes boring—or they give it up completely. The bottom line: Without an ongoing effort to make your partner feel safe expressing the deepest part of themselves, sexual intimacy withers, like a flower deprived of sunlight.

What can we do to prevent sexual intimacy from waning—or restart it after it does?

Try this: Give yourself a grade (from A to F) for the effort you put into creating true intimacy with your partner. Now give yourself a grade for the effort you put into everything else—your job, your children, your social life, and so on. Most people give themselves an A or B for everything else—they'd never forget to pick up their kid at school, or blow off an important work assignment—but the grade they give themselves for creating intimacy tends to be closer to a D or an F.

The first step to restarting sexual intimacy, therefore, is usually to shift your priorities. You have to think of your relationship as the launching pad for everything else you want to achieve in your life, including healthy kids, a good career, the enjoyment of friends, and creative pursuits and hobbies. If your partner is happy, they will support you in what you want to achieve. And there's almost nothing two people can't achieve when they're on the same team. The opposite is also true: You may not realize it, but when the most important relationship in your life is troubled, it acts as a drag on your whole life. Most people privately admit to me, "When I'm fighting with my partner, *nothing* feels right. When we feel close, *everything* feels right."

To be more specific: It is your responsibility to create an "air" of sexual intimacy *all the time*—especially when you're not having sex. It's like a wink or a nod that acknowledges you see your partner as a *sexual* being, that you haven't forgotten that dimension of life. This creates something important: a context where, even if it's not happening right now, sexuality is alive in the relationship. This can take many different forms, and I encourage you to be creative. It could be moments during the day when you touch your partner in a meaningful way, or leave sexy messages for one another. It could be in the tone of voice with which you say, "I love you." Not as though it's an obligation, but as the meaningful statement it should be. Don't just pass your partner in the kitchen; rather, touch them or give them a kiss. These small sexual "injections"—verbal, physical, facial, even energetic—are the lifeblood of intimacy. They also signal to your partner that it's safe for them to respond in a similar way.

Make a commitment to do this—just like when you show up on

time for work: *I'm going to do something today to make my partner feel like a sexually attractive being.*

But what if someone isn't feeling loving or sexually attracted to their partner?

Most relationships will reach the stage where whatever attracted you in the first place has disappeared. That may seem like a serious problem, but in the vast majority of cases, it isn't. For most couples, sexual attraction doesn't literally go away, it just gets buried for all the reasons I mentioned. The important thing is to do something. If you do nothing, it will only get worse. If I can get a person to "act as if" they feel attracted, not only does their partner start to feel closer to them, but they themselves start to feel their attraction returning. As they say in 12-step groups, you have to "fake it 'til you make it."

An Exercise for Reigniting Attraction

I recommend to my patients that they do this exercise with their partner at least once a week before they go to sleep at night. Make sure you won't be interrupted by the phone or the kids, and set a timer for 60 seconds. Then do the following:

1. Stare into each other's eyes. Don't try to read what the other person is thinking or feeling. Instead, even though you're looking at your partner, focus your attention inside of yourself.

2. Visualize the most vulnerable part of yourself. (This is your Shadow, the part of you that you're most embarrassed to expose to your partner. Often, the Shadow will seem scared—it wants love but doesn't trust that the love is real.) Be loving and reassuring to it, the way you would be with a small child who is afraid of the dark.

3. Open your heart and silently visualize bringing your Shadow forward and revealing it to your partner. If you're doing it right, it will require courage, because it'll make you feel a little exposed. Again, do not pay attention to the other person's reaction. The point is to reveal your Shadow without any shame.

4. If you find yourself picking up judgment from the other person, assume it's you judging your own Shadow. Immediately reassure your Shadow—go back to steps 2 and 3. Keep repeating this as many times as you need to.

Do you find that busyness gets in the way of intimacy?

Modern life is *incredibly* demanding. None of us have enough time. But intimacy is more a matter of *energy* than time. The steps I've outlined don't actually take that much time, but they shift the energy of a relationship dramatically. If the message you're sending your partner is consistent—"I actively *see* you and it turns me on"—I doubt you'll have to spend any more time together than you do now...although you might find yourself *wanting* to. And wouldn't that be great?

Have you seen more problems with intimacy since the rise of technology?

Yes, and it's simply because our electronic devices are ubiquitous and give us a convenient way to avoid intimacy. The truth is, intimacy requires effort. And you may not be aware of it, but it also requires courage. Every time you come on to your partner, whether it results in sex or not, you're risking rejection. It's much "safer" to bury yourself in social media, the news, or texting a friend. But in the long run, that destroys the sense of connection relationships thrive on. One more thing: You can't complain about not having enough time for intimacy if you spend hours playing *Candy Crush* every night...

Do you see a connection between your work on the Shadow and attraction?

Yes! The Shadow is a vast and complex subject, but to simplify it, you can think of the Shadow as a part of you—like a separate being living inside you. The Shadow, which was discovered by the psychiatrist Carl Jung, embodies whatever qualities you feel aren't "right"—qualities that endanger your organized, controlled existence; it's messy. You hide the Shadow most of the time—you'd be too embarrassed to let all the world see it—but when free of the need to be "polite" or "appropriate," it comes out.

> *The Shadow, which was discovered by the psychiatrist Carl Jung, embodies whatever qualities you feel aren't "right"—qualities that endanger your organized, controlled existence; it's messy. You hide the Shadow most of the time—you'd be too embarrassed to let all the world see it—but when free of the need to be "polite" or "appropriate," it comes out.*

When you have sex—particularly mind-blowing sex—the Shadow takes over. Meaning the Shadow is the most passionate part of you—intensely sexual and capable of pleasure that's beyond what you normally experience.

For obvious reasons, the Shadow is the key to revitalizing your sex life. Your task is to stay in touch with it whenever you're in the presence of your partner. One way to do that is simply to have an image of your Shadow—and see it in your mind's eye whenever you're with your partner. (Take a moment right now and visualize yourself having ecstatic sex with someone. That image of yourself—free of all inhibition and filled with passion—is what you want to visualize whenever you're around your partner.) You don't have to tell your partner (or anyone else) you're visualizing having sex, but doing so reminds you that you have a sexual self—and that you want it to be present whenever your partner is present. There's an added benefit to this: Every time you visualize your Shadow, you're reminding yourself that you value this most vulnerable part—that you're not going to ignore it even if your partner does. As your Shadow feels more recognized by you, its feelings of sexuality will become more available to you.

And, strangely, your relationship will likely improve as well. People are psychically connected to one another. Your partner may never know you're visualizing your Shadow, but he or she will feel as if there's something you're bringing into the relationship that's exclusive, an energy you share only with each other. The specialness of that experience almost inevitably brings two people closer together.

What if we try all this and our partner still seems uninterested in sex?

That's the time for a serious discussion. Try to find out why your partner is resisting your attempts. Don't threaten or attack; make it safe for them to reveal what's going on. You can give your partner time to think about (or reveal) what's going on, but you also have to send a firm message: "I'm not going to stay in a sexless relationship—I don't mean that as a threat; it's just a fact."

Couples therapy (or individual therapy for the resistant partner) also may help. But the bottom line is that you have to trust your instincts. Do you sense your partner is taking the problem seriously, actually working to unblock themselves? Or are they paying lip service to it without really doing the work?

Are there certain times in a relationship when external factors cause attraction to wane?

On top of the normal waxing and waning of intimacy, these (and other) major life events tend to put a crimp in a couple's sex life:

1. When a child is born.
2. When children reach adolescence, particularly when they start to experience their own sexuality. (A lot of parents find it difficult to have freewheeling sex with each other at the same time they might be discouraging it/confronting the topic with their teens.)
3. When children graduate high school and leave home (empty-nest syndrome).
4. Whenever any other highly stressful event occurs, such as a serious illness or death in the family, a geographical move, or a job dislocation.

These events don't have to destroy intimacy. But when relevant, it's a good idea to identify the risk with your partner and work even harder to sustain intimacy throughout the difficult period. Remember: The imperative in a relationship is to be a team—and since these events tend to put distance between you, you'll have to work harder than usual to stay together in the midst of them.

In your experience, is there one enduring turn-on?
I've been married for thirty-plus years, and what I've found (personally and professionally) is that there's only one enduring turn-on. It's a guaranteed turn-on, but it's not easy.

The one enduring turn-on is *knowing* someone more deeply than anyone else knows them, and allowing them to know you more deeply than anyone else knows you. Not just your good qualities, not the airbrushed persona you project to the world, but everything you hide, including the lost, fallen parts of yourself, your secret insecurities, your vulnerabilities, and everything else you're most deeply ashamed of. To have another human being know those secret, unrevealed parts of you, and gently hold them in his or her heart, is to experience an unusual kind of bliss—the ultimate bliss.

But be honest with yourself: It's really scary to reveal those parts of you; most people will do almost anything to avoid doing so. Which is why we crave quick fixes to turn us on: sex toys, face-lifts, drugs and alcohol, sexual "techniques," and so on. We try to "consume" our way into intimacy. It doesn't work. Real intimacy is an ongoing process of revealing every part of yourself to your partner—especially the parts you'd never reveal to anyone else.

Which leads to an unexpected conclusion: The inner quality that is most important in sustaining intimacy isn't physical attractiveness or sexual prowess; it's bravery.

To paraphrase the writer Anaïs Nin, "One's sex life contracts or expands in proportion to one's courage."

PART TWO
Sexuality

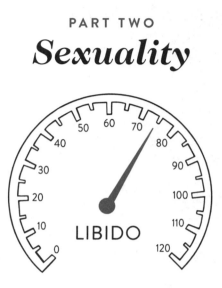

The brilliant Esther Perel (see page 13) points out that sexuality is not just something you do—it's a place you go. "It taps into various parts of you," she says. "It's a language that you express, and you experience." As a culture, we focus a lot on the roots of our sexuality—nature vs. nurture. This obscures the richness of what sexuality truly is, and how intimately tied it is to who we really are, no matter where different aspects of it might originate.

The idea that sexuality *is* our life force—as a number of experts in this section contend—shifts perspective away from specific definitions to an acceptance of a rich, incredibly powerful part of existence. Cultivating our sexuality; celebrating it, as opposed to simply defining it;

awakening, strengthening, exploring, and honoring it, pays off not just in an improved sex life, but in an improved life overall. The more we live in that place Perel talks about, the more we know and fully experience the miracle that is ourselves.

CHAPTER 10

libido: the ebbs and the flows

As anyone who has ever lost her mojo will tell you, the strength of one's libido is subject to some ebbs and flows. In her LA-based practice, clinical psychologist and certified sex therapist Shannon Chavez takes a holistic approach to concerns over swings in libido—exploring potential root causes—from the physical to the emotional. Likewise, our sexual energy affects the person we are in every realm of life, not just inside the bedroom. One of the biggest libido killers—and drains on our overall energy and sex life? Stress, says Chavez. While Chavez is clear that we shouldn't compare our libido to anyone else's—she likens your libido to your fingerprint—it's true that most of us could use more play in life and that it's always a good idea to invest in some TLC for one's own libido.

Keeping Your Libido in Shape

SHANNON CHAVEZ, PSYD

What is libido? How is it different from desire?

Libido is our drive toward pleasure and is connected to arousal and desire. Libido has biological, psychological, and social components influenced by hormones, mood, and our environment. It's all about *energy*. Libido is the source of our life force and creativity. Desire is our motivation toward an object or person. Libido drives desire. Without it, we don't engage in activities that bring us pleasure, which will ultimately affect our health and well-being.

How does libido shape your sexuality?

Libido and sexual response go hand in hand. Some schools of thought refer to libido as the drive or motivation toward sex. When libido is present, there will be urges and the desire to engage in sexual activity or fantasy. Libido can trigger sexual arousal—emotional and physiological changes initiated by the processing of internal or external stimuli—and tends to be an automatic response.

Libido is multifaceted when it comes to our relationship with sexuality, and the causes of ups and downs are related to many different factors. The first factor involves medical, psychological, or physiological changes that may cause libido to go high or low. Though the research is inconclusive, there does seem to be a relationship between hormone levels and sex drive. Common causes of low libido include changes in hormones, childbirth, medication, and birth control. Libido is also connected to our relationship with self and others. Libido can feel low if you are out of touch with your sexuality or with your sexual feelings and desires. A lower libido might relate to negative beliefs and values around sex and associations to sex that are less about pleasure and more about pressure or obligation.

For most individuals, does libido tend to be subject to ebb and flow, or to be more fixed? Are some people just more sexual?

Libido is constantly changing and evolving like most aspects of our sexuality. It can ebb and flow regardless of age, ethnicity, or lifestyle, and affects women who have children as well as those who do not. It affects those who think they are attractive, as well as those who are critical of their appearance. It affects people who are single, coupled, or in open relationships.

There is no norm when it comes to libido, so we shouldn't compare ourselves to others.

There is no norm when it comes to libido, so we shouldn't compare ourselves to others. It is important for everyone to find their "norm" and work toward improvement of overall health and well-being rather than being driven by shame or embarrassment to fit sexual ideals that are not your own.

Another way to think of it: Libido is as unique to everyone as a fingerprint. It is in part programmed at birth and during critical periods throughout our development when the brain is adapting to new sights, sounds, tastes, and touches. (Major periods of development include birth, infancy, childhood, and adolescence.) Every experience we have influences our libido and programs how we respond to receiving and giving pleasure. The good news is that it is possible to recondition our libido and awaken our libidinal energy through positive sexual experiences, intention, sex therapy and treatment, and self-care.

When is libido—either too high or too low—a cause of potential concern? How do you approach libido concerns with patients?

Your libido might feel high or low or even absent altogether. Low libido is a common sexual concern, and most symptoms include lack of interest in and/or desire for sex, difficulty getting and staying aroused, and sexual avoidance. A high libido can be healthy and is a concern only when it leads to out-of-control sexual behaviors and causes distress in the individual. (Again, libido is really personal. There is no good, bad, or normal.)

When working with patients around libido concerns, I always do a thorough sexual health assessment and determine if any of the following factors are present: depression, fatigue, relationship issues, lack of privacy, stress, trauma, fear, anxiety, boredom, or job dissatisfaction.

Regaining a healthy libido is about balance. Often individuals are using up all their libido in one area of life and feeling depleted in another. We help our patients work to balance these areas and create space for sexual self-realization and care, which leads to feeling more sexually alive and aware of one's sexual desire.

In what other ways do you see libido as related to overall energy?

When someone is dealing with libido issues, those issues are usually connected to changes in life, inadequate coping mechanisms, and psychological factors that need to be dealt with. Most people are facing libido killers in day-to-day life: stress, poor diet and nutrition, and mental health concerns such as anxiety and depression. These factors bring drastic changes to energy levels and mood.

Stress is one of the biggest factors connected to libido and one of the most important to fix. If you are stressed and your mind-set is *not enough time*, *not in the mood*, and *not interested*—then the first steps are to create space, practice mindfulness, and move from a state of energy deficit into a state of energy surplus to enable experiences that bring joy, pleasure, and excitement.

Many adults are not getting enough play in life. They are run down by work and not feeling creative or free in other areas of life. Sexual energy is creative energy and is connected to how we express ourselves in all areas of life. Get your libido in shape by staying active, connecting with nature, maintaining a healthy mind and body, and creating sexual experiences that are novel and exciting.

FROM THE GOOPASUTRA
WAYS TO RELAX—SO YOU CAN REALLY GET EXCITED

Stress rarely makes a person feel terribly sexy, notwithstanding the occasional sudden fight-or-flight surge of adrenaline that leads to a steamy encounter. If your work project is late, your fridge is empty, you forgot to call your mom back, the kids won't do their homework, and something's up with the dog—it's nearly impossible to tumble into bed and start to feel something. Here are some ways to get back in touch with your body and dial down your stress level:

- Take a bath full of healing salts and essential oils.
- Focus on your breath. If you've got a mantra or a meditation practice, enter it; if you don't, try thinking *let* as you breathe in, and *go* as you breathe out.
- Exercise. Your blood moves, your cheeks flush, you both get in touch with and feel better about your body…Even taking a walk around the block can do the trick.
- Massage your own feet with lovely body cream.
- Watch—in a focused, calm way—either the clouds, waves, or a lit candle.
- Walk in your garden and run your fingers through the plants you like the scent of—rosemary, black currant, and lavender are especially good for women—and inhale.
- Read a book—not on a screen.

tantric sex

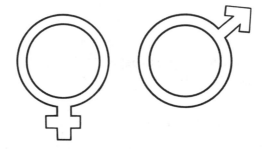

International teacher and relationship counselor Michaela Boehm busts myths about Tantra: Only a small part of the practice actually concerns sex. As Boehm, author of *The Wild Woman's Way*, explains, authentic Tantra is focused on self-improvement and healing, especially on cultivating embodied attention and awareness, which in turn expands our capacity for intimacy with others. When it comes to our intimate relationships, she says that polarity—the tension between masculine energy and feminine energy—or what she calls "Erotic Friction," is key. When the spark goes out in a long-term relationship, Boehm finds it is often because the people in the relationship have naturally become more similar over time. This doesn't mean you should run out and find your opposite—compatibility in a partner is key, and there isn't a guide to finding it. What Boehm presents as the vastly easier option is her Tantra-based road map of principles to increase the polarity between you and your partner, which in turn can spike sexual attraction. But you don't actually have to be in a relationship to find value in understanding how our negative and feminine energies interact (we all have both)—it is illuminating work outside the bedroom as well.

Erotic Friction: Masculine vs. Feminine Energy

MICHAELA BOEHM

What is Tantra, and what is it based in?

The way Tantra is generally presented in the West today is very different from the original ways it was practiced. There are many neo-Tantric schools and paths, most of which focus primarily on the sexual aspect of Tantra and use just a select aspect of its vast philosophy for self-improvement and healing.

The original core teachings of Tantra center around the notion that everything is sacred. Only a small portion of the teachings have anything to do with actual sex; most of the practices focus on embodied attention and awareness, which allows us to connect with ourselves, our partners, and the world at large. Even the most mundane activity can be performed as a sacred act and awaken us deeply.

Many of the Tantric practices teach us how to meet all experiences and sensations fully (good and bad alike), with equal acceptance, and to become deeply sensitive to whatever we are feeling. Subsequently, people are then able to connect with others and their needs and desires more easily, which fosters greater intimacy in general and deeper sexual connection with our chosen partners.

Can everyone benefit from Tantra?

Tantra is for anyone who wants to engage themselves and their partners with deeper attention, sensitivity, and feeling. Regardless of whether someone is alone, starting to date, or wants to rekindle the spark in an existing relationship, the practices center on three distinct aspects that allow for a deeper engagement with oneself and another. The first aspect is intimacy, which can be described as the availability of self through attention, sensitivity, and the ability to fully feel. The second is the ability to connect through the heart with compassion and uncensored love. The third involves the principles of polarity, which enable us to create strong erotic attraction.

Can you really manufacture chemistry?

Yes, you can create attraction and erotic tension. There are principles that create a spark between two partners. A more accurate word would be "polarity," or what is called "Erotic Friction" in my particular Kashmir Shaivism tradition of Tantra.

Most of us rely on the spontaneous, magic moments of "chemistry" occurring naturally. In the beginning of a relationship, there is generally spontaneous erotic attraction, but as the relationship matures, the natural attraction and sexual "hotness" diminish. Thankfully, intimacy is a skill that can be cultivated, practiced, and deepened. Polarity can be learned, generated, and increased as a capacity. With the proper tools, the depth and excitement of sexual engagement will be heightened and cultivated way beyond the initial spark.

How do you see the opposition of masculine energy and feminine energy? How does this opposition affect sexual attraction?

Each human has both masculine and feminine in them. We usually tend to enjoy one aspect more than the other—that's what I call sexual preference.

The feminine in men and women alike enjoys the flow of life and love, revels in the ability to enjoy beauty, nature, textures, colors, and experiences. Fullness is the feminine principle. Sexually speaking, the partner with a feminine essence enjoys the aspects of surrender, dissolution, and being ravished.

The masculine in men and women alike enjoys the forward motion of directed action and purpose, organization, and linear planning. In everyday life, the masculine tends to engage in competition (in business as well as in sports) and focused mental activity, and replenishes best by having "nothing" to do (this could take the form of "zoning out" in front of the TV, having a drink, engaging in sexual activity, or practicing meditation). The masculine principle is emptiness. Sexually speaking, the masculine enjoys the ravishing, taking, penetrating aspect of the erotic play.

Men and women have both traits, but in a polarized (meaning sexually oriented) relationship, one partner takes on the feminine expression and one takes on the more masculine expression; the radical differences in orientation create a strong arc of sexual polarity. The further the "poles" are apart, the stronger the sexual attraction.

In long-term relationships, partners often become very much the same—we start to like the same things, do the same activities, live together, spend much time together. Over time, the couple resonate rather than polarize and hence there is less sexual attraction. But a good relationship fundamentally relies on "sameness." The more a couple agree on common goals, values, activities, and preferences, the better the relationship.

In long-term relationships, partners often become very much the same—we start to like the same things, do the same activities, live together, spend much time together. Over time, the couple resonate rather than polarize and hence there is less sexual attraction.

The good news is that sexual attraction follows principles that can be easily learned and practiced. It is much harder to find a compatible partner than to re-create strong erotic attraction.

What's the key to balancing masculine and feminine aspects?

There are several considerations. As both men and women carry both masculine and feminine within them, the key is to understand that each of those aspects, and their activities, is useful and valid for every human.

Women need decisive ability as much as men need feeling capacity, and vice versa. The important distinction here is that whatever we do most produces the strongest patterns in our bodies. If you prefer the feminine pole of sexual engagement and you spend all day doing masculine activities, your body will not have the skills to effortlessly switch into the soft, receptive, sensual mode you'd prefer to enjoy with your partner. There is no need to malign any aspect of ourselves—the masculine is as important as the feminine; it's just a matter of being facile in both domains. That way we can kick ass in the boardroom and enjoy softness and pleasure in the bedroom.

It's important to examine which bodily patterns are less developed and learn the skills needed to ensure that both aspects are well developed and available. We can then choose pleasure and intimacy as well as decisive action and focus, and make the shift as needed in our lives.

Can you give an example of how someone might increase "Erotic Friction"?

1. Reclaim Your Feminine

If you spend your day in masculine energy but want to set the stage for sex when you get home, you might need to get back into the feminine, or "full" again: Have a glass of wine, take a bath, chat with a friend. Meanwhile, your partner might want to stay in, or get into the masculine: This means that he or she wants to get "empty" or be quiet . . . so if you can, resist the urge to download your partner on your day until you've both had a chance to get into your respective aspects. As you come through the door from the office, let your partner direct you to have a glass of wine or take a bath. Women balk at this, but for sexual tension, it's essential. There needs to be that separation— getting full and getting empty—before coming together again fully charged.

2. Decode the Underlying Dynamic

There was a fascinating study on marriage (published in 2013, but drawing on data from the '90s) that found when men do more or an equal amount of housework, the couples have less sex. Understandably, women felt that the research results undermined an equality decades in the making. So here is the thing: It's all in the framing. With a subtle shift—coming home to a husband who directs you to have a glass of wine while he finishes up dinner prep suddenly sounds quite sexy. The direction—the assumption of the masculine aspect—is a subtle but essential necessity.

3. Learn How to Give Directions

Biologically, women are not inclined to have sex with a man they do not trust—and trust can mean many things. Trust might revolve around competency (i.e., a forgetful, unreliable man is not attractive). Interestingly, in my marriage, and in the marriages of many of my clients, guys are not as good at directions and navigating. I would know my husband was going the wrong way, would suggest he change course, and then be annoyed and turn away from him or pick a fight. It was unattractive all around. Now we have a system in place that is empowering: It empowers me to ensure that we get to where we're supposed to go, and it makes him not look or feel incompetent as a driver. It's very simple: We get in the car, he turns to me, and he tells me to tell him where to go. He is directing me to direct him.

Can other energy meridians affect our sexuality and sexual energy?

In most Eastern healing modalities, there is mention of energy channels or meridians. In my lineage, we look at "channels" as pathways of energy throughout the body. Some of those channels at times become blocked or have restricted flow, which results in physical and/or emotional blocks. Blockages affect the way we experience pleasure and how much we are able to open to intimacy, as well as general vitality and health. Stress, trauma, bad habits, and health conditions are a few reasons why energy might become stagnant.

I teach numerous somatic techniques to free the "flow" within the body, which affects mood, vitality, and the ability to feel sensual and sexual pleasure.

Is there a certain Tantra practice that's good to begin experimenting with?

There are many practices that are easily integrated into everyday life. One of the simplest relational practices is to spend a designated amount of time connecting with each other. As little as five minutes of uninterrupted eye contact and attention can make a huge difference in the domain of intimacy:

Sit across from each other in a comfortable position. Set the timer and begin to connect through eye contact. This might feel strange and induce giggles or discomfort, but there is no need to be serious; just experience whatever arises. You don't have to stare; easy connection and a loving attitude are all it takes. Notice what happens when distractions fall away. You could hold hands or connect through knees and thighs, but see if you can refrain from talking as a means of reducing the habitual ways of avoiding intimacy. Smile or just relax into the eye contact. Once the timer has ended the practice, offer each other a hug or even a formal bow to signify the end. Talk about the experience afterward.

This practice is foundational in becoming more sensitive to internal experiences while connecting to your partner without distraction or established habits. The same principles of focused, uninterrupted attention are easily applied to talk or touch, as well as other sexual activities.

FROM THE GOOPASUTRA
THE SECRET SEX WISDOM OF THE SACRED SNAKE CEREMONY

A lot of what spiritual intimacy teacher Londin Angel Winters helps women do involves getting out of their heads and into their own bodies and divine feminine power. She offers workshops, intensives, coaching sessions, and online courses (some for men, too, alongside her male partner) designed to heal deep-seated wounds, awaken sexual energy in individuals, and deepen intimacy among couples.

The wisdom offered by Winters takes a few different forms, the least conventional being a "sacred snake ceremony." Say what? To the beat of trance-like tunes, Winters demonstrates how to vibe with actual snakes, which she deems subtle energy masters, capable of unlocking a woman's own sensuality and power. Winters sees the movement as a lost art (think ancient temple dances), and explains that snakes are highly sensitive feelers (they can detect infrared heat radiation from warm bodies) and contain some of the oldest DNA on the planet ("They survived extinction!"). Almost everyone who comes for a sacred snake dance (Winters does private dives as well as group parties) is, ahem, nervous at the outset. What's unexpected is how quickly you become comfortable—and even at peace—with Winters's four snakes on your body: a (big!) lavender albino ball python named Snakleton; a Bolivian short-tailed boa named

BoJack; a baby Colombian boa called Primo (whose parents are both thirteen feet); and Vincent, a female jaguar carpet python named after the favorite poet of Winters (Edna St. Vincent Millay). It sounds crazy, but there's something both calming and electrifying about feeling the snakes move effortlessly over your body, tuning you into sensation and, really, just being present in your skin. You leave feeling very alive—and not afraid of snakes at all.

CHAPTER 12

owning your sexual power

Sexuality is a great source of personal pleasure and inner power, but, for a host of reasons—including societal misconceptions and pressures as well as long-standing narratives that are perpetuated by the media (as well as everyone else)—girls and women often internalize the message that projecting sexuality is more important than feeling it. This injustice is part of what clinical and cultural sexologist, social worker, and sexuality educator Zelaika S. Hepworth Clarke explores. Clarke's research on empowerment, sexual-sensual liberation, and the effects of colonialism have brought her around the world and helped her develop a nuanced, layered understanding of different ways of feeling and experiencing sexual pleasure and eroticism, both within and outside of traditionally patriarchal societies. Here, she illuminates more perspectives and shares her own empowering take on how we can tap into our sexual power and access pleasure without shame.

The Devouring Vagina and Other Ways of Embracing Sexuality

ZELAIKA S. HEPWORTH CLARKE, PHD

What is the concept of "the devouring vagina"?

I first read about the "devouring vagina" in a piece from the feminist scholar Nkiru Nzegwu on osunality, or African sensuality-sexuality, that affirms that feeling sexual pleasure and being erotic is normal and natural. She explores this idea of the devouring vagina, which is based on the imagery during hetero sex of the penis disappearing, or being devoured—alluding to the strength and power of the vagina.

In Western narratives, the penis is usually seen as dominant, but in this particular paradigm, an agency, or activeness, is assigned to the vagina, while a measure of passivity is assigned to the penis.

In Western narratives, the penis is usually seen as dominant, but in this particular paradigm, an agency, or activeness, is assigned to the vagina, while a measure of passivity is assigned to the penis. The penis is enveloped, swallowed, and made to disappear; the withdrawing of the penis is seen as an act of resistance from being pulled in or reswallowed by the demanding vagina.

This allowed me to consider a narrative that speaks to a different perspective. It opened up a way of knowing that sex does not have to revolve around a penis. It made me aware of all these scripts I've potentially internalized. In our language, we say things like "beat it up," "hit it," "banging out," "smashed," "wham," "screw," even "losing" someone's virginity, or virginity being "taken away." Those are all colloquialisms that have violent undertones. It's a narrative I don't find very empowering.

The body is very powerful in subjectively understanding pleasure. We often say, "This is *giving* me pleasure," rather than recognizing the body's interpretation of different stimuli as pleasure. It's powerful to shift our views of where we're placing emphasis. Genitals aren't the only sex organ—our minds, our skin, and other parts of the body also derive pleasure; sexuality can be a full-body experience in which pleasure is derived through different senses, whether sound, taste, smell, or touch.

How can we access pleasure without shame?

When I started thinking about where my own shame came from, I realized it was a product of judgmental value systems that had caused me to think I was doing something wrong, or that there was a better, moral way to be human. When I was studying the African/Brazilian spiritual tradition of candomblé, I learned there was no such thing as sin—sin was thought of as a white male concept used to control people. Consider seriously for a moment that perhaps sin doesn't exist, or that what we have been told is bad may not need to have so much judgment. With that, I opened up different ways of knowing myself, and that completely shifted my shame.

There are a lot of negative messages around sex, pleasure, eroticism, and the way we're supposed to relate to people. (I had been told that sex was dirty.) The messages are very scripted and controlled by hegemonic forces—generally able-bodied, white, Western, usually Christian, well-to-do. When I'm able to think critically about where these scripts are coming from, and if I've internalized any of them, the question becomes, Is this really helpful and beneficial to me? Is this an empowering approach?

Also, a lot of the narratives happen not to be written by women, even if they're about women. Take menstruation, for example: There's a lot of negativity around it—that it's painful, inconvenient, gross—when there are other nonjudgmental approaches available. I think radical self-acceptance really helped me deal with shame—but also to question all the narratives that have been prescribed that could lead to shame, too.

Therefore, accessing pleasure without shame is about letting go of the messages and conditioning we've internalized that almost make us forget the power we have inside us. My shame dissipates when I'm not judgmental, but I have to reprogram my brain to be able to imagine what it's like.

What are some alternative ways of understanding sexuality that you've encountered historically?

The word "heterosexuality" wasn't even in the dictionary until after 1901, so we're talking about a fairly new way of looking at this concept in a specific way. Sexuality was probably perceived as something very different throughout most of time, which is also true for how we understand gender. The scholar María Lugones first made the claim that gender is a colonial imposition; I think there's a lot to say for that. Many Indigenous languages don't need pronouns. They're gender-neutral and not binary. That thinking can heavily impact the way we understand the world and ourselves.

How do you tap into sexuality's full power?

Be open-minded to who you are and what your desires are. Power looks different to different people. People express themselves as powerful beings in different ways. I think a lot of marginalized populations have been conditioned to think they have no power. For me, sexuality and understanding the power of sexuality come with self-knowledge and self-acceptance—which I tap into by practicing mindfulness—in other words, letting go and being in the present here and now.

Not everything has to be separate. I was taught that spirituality and sexuality are completely different and they don't overlap, but I've since experienced other cultures and traditions like Tantra where sexuality and spirituality are very much intertwined. What gives you pleasure; what makes you feel passion? There's power in knowing pleasure.

What can we do when we feel disempowered?

I start by shifting my attitude toward gratefulness and appreciation. Instead of thinking about what I don't have or what I want, I think about what I do have; sometimes it's just being grateful to be able to breathe, grateful for the sun, grateful that I live on earth, grateful for water, grateful to be human. Putting things in perspective is helpful. Letting go of judgment toward myself is also helpful. I move toward positive affirmation and start taking myself on as a lover. Asking: *Why am I saying this to myself if I wouldn't say it to my lover? Why am I being so mean to myself? Do I tell myself "I love you, you look beautiful"?* Develop a relationship with yourself and be patient.

This can be hard when we're not seeing representations of our beauty and sexuality around us—what can we do?

We need critical thinking. I have to develop ways of being able to identify, "Wow, that's photoshopped," or "That's not even real." You may have to go on a media diet for a bit, or decrease or change how you're getting that type of information. We stress visuals and aesthetics, but I think real beauty often emanates from places that can't be seen, and there are aspects of beauty we haven't been told about yet.

What does the term "sex-positive" really mean?

For me, being sex-positive celebrates the diversity of pleasurable experiences and respects self-determined sexiness. One of my favorite rules in sexuality education for creating a safer environment is: "Don't yuck someone's yum." Everyone is different; everyone has their own erogenous zones and ways they experience sexuality and pleasure, pain, and eroticism. Being sex-positive includes the affirmation of desire without shame.

Desire looks different in different cultures, so we have to be careful not to project onto others our own positivity or what it means for us. A lot of times we'll say, "Oh, wow, sex should be orgasmic. Sex should be juicy." Some cultures and people don't prefer it that way, which can still be affirmed and respected. It's about being less judge-y and more accepting (with the exception of cases involving harm to other people and issues of consent)—practicing compassion with yourself and others.

I like to think about my "innerverse," or inner universe, being open to the diversity within myself, and the fact that things change with time. What we find pleasurable at one time in our lives may be different from what we find pleasurable at other times; even our desire can be situational. I love the concept of "the pluriverse"—multiple realities existing simultaneously without hierarchy, even with a contradictory understanding. Whether it's the devouring vagina or a very different phallocentric narrative around sex, one doesn't have to undermine the other. They both can exist.

FROM THE GOOPASUTRA
OUR FIRST TIME

We polled GOOP HQ with the question: What was your first time like? In the responses, we heard echoes of the ingrained language that Clarke points out:

- "We were on a dark tennis court after breaking into a pool club, in a rampant last-ditch effort after figuring out we had nowhere else to go. It was a sticky, humid summer night. The sex was anticlimactic—figuratively and literally. It was awkward, quick, and bloody."

- "Sloppy? I was drunk; he was drunk. So many years later, and we wonder why anyone makes a big deal about it."

- "With my first boyfriend, at the age of seventeen. We promised to wait until six months of dating. I appreciate that he was a good boyfriend, very sweet and caring, and we were each other's firsts. It felt very safe. (I wasn't in touch with myself enough yet to find it very pleasurable, but I did soon.) I met my friend at the gym afterward, and I remember thinking in step class, 'No one here has any idea I just had sex for the first time, do I look different? I don't look or feel different.'"

- "Fast!"

- "It was on Valentine's Day when I was sixteen with my boyfriend of a year. We didn't know what we were doing, and it was painful and not enjoyable. We tried again in the morning and it was a bit better, but nothing to write home about."

- "I think the best part about my first time was my outfit from that night. Faux-fur vest and combat boots. I was in college and I'm not sure if the guy knew it was my first time. Before having sex, I had felt a lot of pressure to lose my virginity; it was kind of a relief once it happened."

- "With my high school sweetheart in the back of my car! So cliché, but it was after a trip to NYC and we couldn't wait until we got home, and we likely didn't have an empty house to go to."

- "I lay on my back and we kissed for a little. The sex was uncomfortable and it was done in like five minutes. I was excited before and during, but it turned out to be not as amazing as I thought afterwards."

- "Pretty textbook: high school boyfriend while his parents were out of town."

- "Terrible. Both our parents were really strict, so we were in a car. Let's just say: Nothing about it worked."

- "It was with my first boyfriend. I was a virgin and he wasn't, so it was up to me when I wanted to do it. I kept putting it off, until one day we were grocery shopping and I just said very casually, 'Let's get condoms.' I still remember how quickly his face lit up. We hurried home (granted, this was in high school so it was his parents' house), snuck quietly to the basement, and positioned ourselves on the couch. From what I remember, it took about thirty seconds, *The Wizard of Oz* was on TV, and I had to watch lions and tigers and bears dancing around in the background. I remember thinking, 'So that was sex,' afterward. Could have been better, could have been worse."

- "Underwhelming. I was seventeen and embarrassed to be inexperienced with my rather experienced partner. I didn't tell him it was my first time, and I am not sure if he knew or not (or how experienced he really was, in hindsight). I remember thinking that I was going to feel different afterward, or that something was going to change; I remember looking in the mirror in the following days wondering if I was different, but I wasn't. Sounds like a cliché. I was kind of a cliché."

- "I was a freshman in college, and essentially gave my virginity to the first guy I could find. I wanted to be rid of it, as I had absorbed a negative perception from my major crush in high school that I wasn't as desirable as a virgin. I don't regret this choice. The relative anonymity of it allowed me to connect deeply with what I wanted and how my body felt without worrying much about how much my partner was being pleased. I don't think I was selfish, but it definitely encouraged me to explore my sexuality more than if I'd been in love."

- "I was seventeen, neither of us knew what we were doing, and it was just okay."

- "Quick. But, I was in love with my boyfriend and thought I was going to marry him (at sixteen!)."

getting kinky

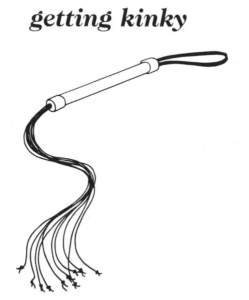

The terms "fetish" and "kink" are often misused, and that doesn't make the topics, which tend to be shrouded in shame, any easier to talk about. For a long time, journalist Jillian Keenan—who wrote the memoir *Sex with Shakespeare* in part about her own fetish for spanking and discipline—thought there was something wrong with her, until she learned to both accept and embrace it. Here, she unpacks the (debated) difference between a fetish (innate, lifelong sexual orientation) and a kink (an interest or preference), and how to open up to the idea of—and have fun with—either.

Exploring a Fetish or a Kink

JILLIAN KEENAN

What is a kink?

A kink is an unconventional sexual interest or preference. Some kinks focus on activities, such as bondage or spanking. Others emphasize identities, like age play or puppy play; or relationship dynamics, like dominant/submissive. There are also kinks that fixate on objects, materials, or body parts, such as diapers, latex, or feet. In many cases, these interests fall under the umbrella known as BDSM: bondage and discipline, dominance and submission, sadism and masochism.

What's the difference between a fetish and a kink?

Fetishists and kinksters aren't homogeneous, and these terms are evolving and hotly debated. Ask three different members of your community to define them, and you'll probably get five different answers!

But in my opinion, a kink is any nonnormative sexual interest that exists alongside sex. It's possible to choose to experiment with kink, or to discover a preference for it later in life. Kink is a preference, analogous to any other: Sometimes an interest fades or is supplanted by a newer interest over time, and sometimes it lasts a lifetime.

On the other hand, a fetish (or paraphilia, to use the clinical term) is an innate, unchosen, and lifelong sexual orientation. Rather than being a component of a person's sexual identity, a fetish is its fixed core—and, like any other sexual orientation, it isn't a choice. Its prominence may ebb and flow with the day-to-day variations of life, but the fact that a fetishist is fundamentally fixated on something not typically recognized as "sex" will not change.

To simplify a bit, if you think about conventional sex when you masturbate, you're probably vanilla. If you masturbate to nontraditional activities that ultimately revolve around sex, you're probably kinky. And if you sexually obsess about one specific thing that has absolutely nothing to do with mainstream definitions of "sex," you're probably a fetishist.

How has your fetish informed your life?

A fetish for spanking and discipline has been at my core for as long as I can remember. In other words, spanking occupies the place in my life that sex occupies in the lives of most people. Even as a toddler, I was obsessed with any reference to punishment—especially corporal punishment. While my friends gossiped about steamy sex scenes from *Dawson's Creek*, I was secretly obsessed with things like the disciplinary paddling scene from *Dead Poets Society*.

> *While my friends gossiped about steamy sex scenes from* Dawson's Creek, *I was secretly obsessed with things like the disciplinary paddling scene from* Dead Poets Society.

I knew this was unusual, and for a long time I felt tremendous fear and shame. I thought something was wrong with me—and conventional psychiatry, which stigmatized my fixation as a mental illness, didn't help. It was only as an adult, when I met other fetishists online and in person, that I fully embraced my orientation for the healthy and natural identity it is.

What's the best way to start exploring a fetish or a kink?

Get online! Every fetish and kink has an online community, and exploring on the internet can be a less intimidating way to connect with new friends, share stories, and discover that you're not alone. (I will never forget the amazing moment when I realized that almost every spanking fetishist goes through a phase in childhood where he or she compulsively looks up words like "spanking" and "punishment" in the dictionary: I had thought I was the only one!) After that, the first steps into the off-line fetish communities can be nerve-racking, but I promise: The decision to connect with people who understand and share your identity may be one of the most rewarding decisions of your life. Just be safe, okay?

Has your fetish evolved/changed since you started exploring it?

My comfort level with my fetish has changed. For decades, I couldn't even say the word "spanking" out loud—it was too overwhelming! I was terrified that merely saying the word would spill all my secrets. But getting involved in the fetish community and making friends with people who share my experience has made me feel, for the first time, what I had never felt before: normal.

How should you approach introducing your kink or fetish to your partner?

If you're ready to share your own kink or fetish with your partner: awesome! I admire your courage and honesty, and I hope your partner will, too.

Be patient. This will most likely take time. When I first outed myself to my vanilla fiancé (now husband), I imagined that finally sharing my big secret would be a magic bullet. It wasn't. That first disclosure was merely the beginning of a process of mutual honesty and exploration that took years and continues to this day. Don't expect your partner to magically understand right away. You'll have to answer uncomfortable questions, explain embarrassing things, and probably experience moments of disappointment. Hang in there—the chance to finally be yourself is worth it.

How should you navigate a partner's kink or fetish?

If a partner shares a nonmainstream sexual interest or identity with you, congratulations! That means he or she loves and trusts you enough to be honest about something that is, in many cases, very frightening. Fetishists and kinksters experience a lot of shame and stigma from pop culture, conventional psychiatry, and even the law, so if your partner is scared, please don't minimize the validity of that feeling. (Phrases like "It's no big deal" don't help; the courage it takes to disclose a stigmatized sexual interest or orientation is a big deal, and not something we should minimize.) Ask questions, read books on the subject, and keep an open mind. You might discover that your partner's revelation brings an exciting and meaningful degree of intimacy to your relationship. But feel free to take it slowly: Your comfort level matters, too.

How can we work to unpack the feelings of shame in this realm?

A lot of stigma comes from the mistaken idea that fetishes and kinks are manifestations of mental illness or a response to childhood trauma. Rest assured, they are not. In fact, a 2013 study published in the *Journal of Sexual Medicine* found that BDSM practitioners actually scored better on many indicators of mental health. (This is likely because active BDSM practitioners have gone through the difficult psychological process it takes to acknowledge, accept, and embrace desires and identities that fall outside the mainstream, and not because kinksters are inherently healthier than anyone else.) As long as your sexual identity and practice is consensual, responsible, and risk-aware, it is healthy, natural, and beautiful.

sexual energy

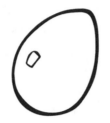

We've long been obsessed with clean-beauty guru, healer, and actress Shiva Rose's naturalist/activist take on life that she reflects on her website, The Local Rose, not to mention her handmade, spirit-infused skin and body treatments. Rose introduced us to the ancient sexual practice of the jade egg one afternoon when she offered to come by and show us how to use one.

Here, Rose explains how the jade egg (and more) helped her connect to her own sexual energy at a point in her life when she needed a reset; and she makes the compelling case that sexual energy is not something to cordon off in the bedroom, but rather a source of energy, power, and confidence that is essential to life.

The Most Powerful Force in the Universe

SHIVA ROSE

In what ways does sexual energy impact the rest of our well-being?

Sexual energy is basically our chi or life force. If it is stagnant and not flowing, our overall well-being, creativity, and health are impacted. This has been common knowledge in Eastern traditions for eons: The Chinese medical tradition, as well as the yogic traditions of India, have always utilized specific exercises, meditations, herbs, kriyas, and practices to get the sexual energy (kundalini) flowing.

> *Sexual energy is what has led us to be here on the earth, to be born, to be created—therefore, it is the most powerful force in the universe.*

Sexual energy is what has led us to be here on the earth, to be born, to be created—therefore, it is the most powerful force in the universe. Sexual energy that is freed up and flowing increases joy, empowerment, bliss, strength, and compassion. You can harness and channel your sexual energy toward various aspects of your life: loving a partner, creating a business, enhancing your spiritual practices. Tools such as qigong, kundalini yoga, meditation, yoni egg exercises, being in nature, touching others, basking in sensual moments, and self-love rituals (to name a few) help us to boost this energy flow and use it to heal.

How does strengthening the vagina affect our overall well-being?

Our willpower, strength, life force, and chi all emanate from the pelvic region. If that area is compromised, then so is our life. The ancient wisdom of the Chinese Taoists is now being rediscovered: Using a jade egg can be a powerful, transformative practice. When you awaken your yoni, you awaken your sexual power, your inner strength, your will, your orgasm, and your life.

How do you do it—is the focus physical, mental, or both?

The yoni egg practice combines mental, physical, and spiritual exercises to reconnect us to this source of chi.

When you first begin and insert the egg, start by just feeling it within the walls of the yoni. You do this lying down on your back, in a sacred ritual that further enhances the experience.

Imagine the energy being created in the yoni, then imagine carrying that energy like a star throughout the body. As with any practice, setting an intention and being in the moment activate the experience further. Chi flows where attention goes.

How did you first connect with your own sexual energy in a deeper way?

When I got divorced eight years ago, I felt I needed to start over and re-create my life. I began practicing kundalini yoga on a consistent basis, and that was my entry into using my sexual—or kundalini—energy to further my life. My kundalini yoga practice led me to discover the jade egg, and once I realized that I was dissociated from my pelvic region, I began to work hard on reclaiming it. By beginning to honor that sacred space within us, we can begin to heal ourselves and become whole.

How did your relationship with your pelvic region evolve into where you are now?

I now feel regions inside my yoni that were once numb. I feel more vibrant and energized, regardless of whether or not I have a lover at the time. My relationship with myself is much deeper, which seems to attract more passion and abundance.

What are signals that one's sexual energy is off?

Strong indications include low libido, lack of lubrication, hormonal issues, not enjoying sex, feeling uncreative, feeling apathetic, experiencing victim mentality, feeling old, numbness, back issues, not being able to have orgasms, urinary incontinence, and depression. The problem can also be related to more subtle issues, like just not being in touch with that energy or that area. I tell people it's like having a room in a beautiful house that's empty, void of any energy, and not being used. It is time then to open the doors to that room, add a table, add a vase with wildflowers in it, raise the window, and allow the wind to clear the area, play some music, and then dance in the room. Feel it becoming alive and full of love.

What should be the first step toward rebalancing our energy?

To begin a relationship with this deepest part of ourselves, we must first acknowledge the fact that we have been avoiding it. Sit quietly, go inward, and begin a dialogue with your inner sanctum, your inner world, your yoni. Tell her that you are sorry for ignoring her all these years, and thank her for all the beautiful creations she is capable of and has brought to you so far. Rub oil on your breasts, rub oil on your belly, rub oil on your yoni. Bathe it in light, beauty, and love. Create a daily relationship with the part of you that is capable of creating life and giving life.

In what ways does sexual energy change over time, and/or with partners?

Sexual energy over time can become stronger and more powerful. It takes work like anything worthwhile, but with daily practice, it will become a way of life that will continue to flow and give.

Partners grow together and reach even deeper places of intimacy and love when they agree to dive in together. Practices like Tantra, in particular, often lead to a deeper and sweeter union.

CHAPTER 15

the art of open relationships

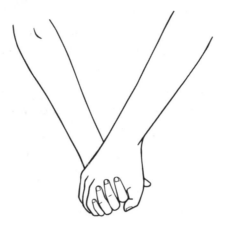

Open relationships might best fall under the category of "To each his or her own." While clearly not for everyone, there are couples for whom monogamy doesn't do it and both partners are happy, and consent, to open up the relationship. If you think this would be insanely complex to navigate, others agree—we asked a social psychologist and faculty affiliate of the Kinsey Institute, Justin Lehmiller, whose work focuses on casual sex, sexual fantasy, and sexual health, to take us through the ground rules of open relationships.

What to Consider Before You Open or Close It

JUSTIN LEHMILLER, PHD

What do you think of open relationships?

I'm a proponent of people making the relationship decisions that are right for them. If you want a monogamous relationship, that's great. But if you want an open relationship or another type of consensually nonmonogamous relationship instead, that's great, too. What the science suggests is that different kinds of relationships work better for different kinds of people. I encourage people to find the kind of relationship that works well for them.

What should you consider before getting into an open relationship?

One of the key considerations is whether you have the right personality for it; these relationships aren't for everyone. According to research, there are at least four personality traits that are relevant when it comes to being in a consensually nonmonogamous relationship.

The first is your sociosexual orientation, which refers to the degree to which you separate sex from emotion. People who have what we call an unrestricted sociosexual orientation are more comfortable with casual sex and don't necessarily need to be close to someone to sleep with them; by contrast, those with what we call a restricted orientation think that sex and love always go together. Not surprisingly, unrestricted folks are more likely to enter open relationships because they're just more suited to them.

Second, people with an insecure attachment style—that is, people who have abandonment issues—don't tend to be as happy in nonmonogamous relationships, which makes sense because they're probably more prone to jealousy.

Two other traits linked to greater happiness in an open relationship are being erotophilic, or having very positive attitudes toward sex;

and being a sexual sensation seeker, or having a preference for thrilling and risky sexual activities.

What all of this tells us is that if you're considering whether an open relationship is right for you, the one dictum you need to remember is "Know thyself."

Are there ground rules that you recommend everyone set?

Open relationships vary dramatically in terms of the specific rules and boundaries negotiated between the partners. What's important is to make sure that it's what you and your partner(s) actually want. Don't do it because you're feeling pressured to do so or because you've somehow convinced yourself that it's a "more evolved" way of having relationships. It's also important to have strong and open communication between the partners and to clearly establish what is and isn't permitted in terms of behavior, sexual and otherwise. For example, are you allowed to have only one-night stands, or is it okay to have an ongoing friend with benefits with whom you have both a sexual relationship and a friendship? It's also important to keep in mind that you don't have to dive right into a completely open relationship—you might want to open it to a limited extent, see how things go, and revise/update the rules later on as you discover what does and doesn't work well.

When it comes to maintaining trust, you need to have some level of trust to begin with, but you also need to establish rules that are realistic and that are going to make you feel secure; otherwise, any trust you have will probably erode pretty quickly.

How do you maintain trust?

When it comes to maintaining trust, you need to have some level of trust to begin with, but you also need to establish rules that are realistic and that are going to make you feel secure; otherwise, any trust you have will probably erode pretty quickly.

Some couples have a full disclosure policy, in which they reveal all the details of their encounters to each other. For some people, this level of communication is necessary for building feelings of security and trust. Others, however, might not want all that detail and might even find it to be threatening, preferring a "Don't ask, don't tell" approach instead. In this case, trust builds differently, accumulating through experience: Though you and your partner might be doing your own thing sexually, you keep coming home to each other. The more experience you have with this, the more confident you'll feel that your partner isn't going to leave.

Can an open relationship be closed and then reopened?

It's possible to close a relationship after you've opened it—and it's also possible to open it up again after closing it. Open relationships are fluid in the sense that the rules can be renegotiated and revised as many times as desired.

We know from research that despite all the effort and care people in open relationships put into establishing rules, many end up breaking those rules. This is because when people make rules about sexual behavior, they tend to do so in a calm, rational state. However, when we're sexually aroused, we aren't always calm and rational—to the contrary, our decision-making ability is impaired and we become more willing to engage in risky behaviors, sexually and otherwise. This may lead us to do things we later regret, such as breaking rules and agreements with a partner. What's important is for you and your partner to feel as though you can disclose rule violations and find a way to deal with them appropriately. In some cases, this might mean temporarily closing the relationship while you figure out a new set of rules.

What do you do if you want to be in an open relationship and your partner doesn't, or vice versa?

An open relationship shouldn't be foisted upon someone who doesn't desire it, because that's not going to turn out well. In cases where couples disagree over whether to open the relationship or not, there are a few options. One is to determine whether there's a mutually agreeable way of adding some novelty and excitement to the relationship that will satisfy the partner who wants to be open without threatening the partner who desires it to be closed. This could take any number of forms, depending on the partners' comfort levels, from watching pornography together to visiting sex shops and strip clubs together to experimenting with sexual role-playing and sex toys. Consulting a sex or relationship therapist might also help. If these things don't work and the partners remain at a sexual impasse, they need to decide whether the relationship is good enough otherwise to continue, or if they would be more content calling it quits so that each of them is free to begin relationships that are more suited to their sexual and romantic needs.

FROM THE GOOPASUTRA
PLAIN EFFING VANILLA

Just because we know about and are open to a new level of variety in terms of human sexual experience doesn't mean plain old vanilla sex—whatever that might mean to you as an individual or couple—doesn't feel fantastic. "When it comes to hot sex, the focus needs to be on pleasure—and that is defined individually," says certified clinical sexologist Eric G. Schneider, MEd, DMin, and a PhD candidate in human sexuality. If doing your same-old-thing favorite routine is still your favorite thing, and your partner feels the same way, don't let the culture of sexual athleticism and achievement (porn, etc.) make you feel like something's wrong. "Keep bringing your focus back to pleasure," says Schneider.

good porn

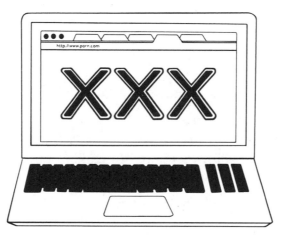

For many of us, porn is a sexist, relationship-wrecking pleasure killer that enforces impossible body standards—and really has no basis in reality whatsoever. But are these qualities inherent to pornography itself? Adult filmmaker Erika Lust says no—she points out that like any medium, porn can be made and used positively and negatively. What's more is that she's set out to prove the point by directing indie-quality pornography films, from the female gaze, in which women are not passive, but pursue their own desires, and men are not reduced to machines, simply hammering away. In order to be sexy, Lust maintains that porn needs a relatable context, an actual narrative, and that the characters need to be sexual collaborators—which is nothing like the majority of the hilariously ludicrous scenarios that play out in mainstream porn (the last time one of our cars broke down on the side of the road, it didn't end in a blow job to a stranger who saved the day . . .).

In one of her film series, called XConfessions, Lust actually bases plots on real fantasies that people submit.

Here, Lust shares what can make porn ethical and orgasm-inducing—and where you can find said porn. (PS: If you're interested in making your own X-rated film at home, Lust has a whole guide to it, titled *Let's Make a Porno*.)

Redefining Porn

ERIKA LUST

How did you get into porn?

Like many young adults, I wanted to explore my sexuality. I was intrigued by pornography, but I was disappointed when I actually watched some films. They were ugly, and the behavior toward women was so degrading and violent sometimes (nothing quite like today's mainstream porn—now it's mostly absurd). I felt aroused physically but I had an uneasy feeling. I could not understand it. It was basically men having sex with women and women engaging in sex for men, and all the scenes were stripped of intimacy, context, and cinematography. Everything I watched was done with such a narrow view of sexuality and lacked sexual intelligence.

At Lund University in Sweden, I studied political science, feminism, and sexuality. I'd always been a movie freak and a lover of creativity and beauty, and after graduating, I moved to Barcelona and started studying filmmaking. I read Linda Williams's book *Hard Core: Power, Pleasure, and the "Frenzy of the Visible,"* and it became clear to me that porn was not "only porn." It was a discourse on sexuality.

I did not agree with the statement on sexuality and gender roles that the mainstream was portraying, and I wanted to create an alternative to a specific type of male gaze that is insidious in mainstream porn. The majority of content out there is laughably unrelatable to female viewers.

(Despite what we're led to believe, women have an active sexuality, too.) I wanted to create adult cinema that reflected my values, my gaze. I started to direct adult movies that I would like myself and that I thought other women and men looking for something fresh, erotic, sensual, and actually sexy would also like. From there, Erika Lust Films grew.

Why do you think porn is such a big piece of people's sex lives and sex education?

We live in a society where sex has been commodified to sell just about anything, from burgers to deodorant. Sexual images have become commonplace, and the increasing prevalence of porn is an extension of that. On top of this, the internet has made accessing explicit images of sex in an inconspicuous way a lot easier and, in most cases, free. One-third of all internet traffic is estimated to be pornography.

We live in a society where sex has been commodified to sell just about anything, from burgers to deodorant.

People have always enjoyed watching sex because it can be fun and pleasurable. Watching porn isn't the problem. Here's what is: Young people are naturally curious about sex, and because of a lack of decent sex education, many turn to the easily accessible porn online way before having real sex. The vast majority of this porn is not designed to be realistic, so teens (and adults) often develop warped expectations that have a huge effect on their sexual behavior.

What role do you see porn playing in a healthy sex life? For someone who has never watched porn, what could it add?

Pornography as a medium can be made and used positively or negatively, in the same way as anything else. Adult cinema that presents people as subjects and sexual collaborators (not objects), offers diversity, represents all the different parts of society, enables people to see themselves in those films, and opens their minds. Apart from being fun to watch, explicit films can be used as a tool for sexual liberation and education. For many viewers, alternative adult cinema helps them celebrate their sexuality and encourages them to be empowered by sex.

Quality erotic films, therefore, can be a wonderful addition in the bedroom. Used properly, they stimulate you and push the boundaries of your own taboos, showing you new experiences and spicing up your sex life by bringing your own fantasies to the forefront. Watching can increase confidence in the bedroom for men and women, as well as electrify the atmosphere and introduce ideas for different role-plays or sexual practices—the possibilities are endless.

Also, watching good adult cinema for masturbation may help someone get to know their body, what they really enjoy and want from a sexual partner, as well as introduce more ways to self-pleasure.

Why is so much porn so bad?

For a long time, watching porn has been touted as a male experience, and it's a cycle: The vast majority of mainstream porn is tacky and ugly, made by one group of people—mostly white, heterosexual men who are comfortable dishing out the same, repetitive films—and often perpetuates very violent and dangerous images of sex, sexuality, and men and women. And it's worked for them.

The internet has completely disrupted the industry, and the free availability of porn everywhere puts further pressure on the production companies and performers to stand out; more and more extreme and ridiculous scenes that have nothing to do with real sex are being produced to that end. I think production companies—especially in comparison to the adult films that were made in the '70s—have forgotten the passion, the intimacy, the touching, and the pursuit of real pleasure in sex, and thus have taken some of the humanity out of it. There is no foreplay, no caressing; performing oral sex on a woman is practically nonexistent. They are focused on only anatomy, genitalia, or body parts bashing against each other. Male pleasure is the ultimate goal—the scene typically unfolds through the male gaze and the cumshot seems to be mandatory to end the scene. The female character is being used to satisfy others, not herself. There are many categories with varied tags and labels that cater to every whim and fetish imaginable, but in the end, it is all the same: just body parts served up in different variations.

That is the reason there are fewer female viewers of mainstream porn—because women in general don't want to deal with porn that is completely neglecting their pleasure on the screen.

The porn industry is also rife with racism. Not only are the films marketed with racialized language, but the sexual content often relies on racist stereotypes as a motive, which dehumanizes the performers. On top of all this, the pay disparity is outrageous. The problem is that porn, unlike other media, often sidesteps scrutiny because we're unwilling to talk about it in public.

What do you think the fix is?

To disrupt the cycle, more women and people of color have to be introduced at the production level. This would bring a healthier, more sex-positive perspective—a willingness to show an authentic representation of human sexuality, where people can explore their sexuality without feeling degraded, marginalized, or guilty. There needs to be relatable context, a narrative, and a connection between characters that are equal to one another. In these quality films, women and men are sexual collaborators. Male characters are human beings, not machines. Women have their own sexuality, and they are not passive objects exclusively focused on pleasuring men; women have a voice in the story and they seek their own desires. There is a mutual exchange of pleasure and respect, and consent is always paramount. All these elements make pornography more realistic and add to its eroticism and arousal.

But thinking bad porn will cease to exist altogether is like thinking that fast food will no longer exist, or that sugar will be prohibited in processed foods like cereal.

How do you define ethical porn?

Ethical porn results when there are proper working conditions for cast and crew; it's about the values the content will transmit; it's quality over quantity. It's caring the same way an organic restaurant cares about their ingredients and cooking process, or how an organic fashion brand cares about the cotton production process.

In my company, every shooting includes a welcoming atmosphere, multiple breaks—and food. My team is present in person and visible online—we have nothing to hide. This seems normal, but in the adult industry, it's not as common as you might think. (Try to find a name or a face on pornhub.com or blacked.com.) Our performers know exactly what will happen on-set and are paid and treated well, and, most importantly, they are not objectified or disembodied. The sex is contextualized with characters and plot, and the entire body of the performers can be seen, not just anatomical shots.

In my films, the performers are all over twenty-one. I make sure they want to perform sex on-camera, and I make sure they know the consequences that entails. Mainstream porn has the tendency to alienate its viewers, so inclusivity is key. I try to work with people of different races, ages, and body types, as this depicts the diversity found in real life.

How much improvisation is there vs. scripted writing typically?

There's a scripted plot and dialogue—I take as much care in writing scripts as any indie film director. I tell the performers what kind of sex I'm looking for, but I try not to direct the sex at all. I want performers to be themselves and have sex as they would at home—to do what feels natural and pleasurable for them. I make sure they are able to talk to each other about their limits, likes, and dislikes before shooting. I don't tell them, "Put your leg here," or "Move your arm there," or "Do five different positions and show me your butthole!" I am not interested in that. Performers have a better time when the sex is more natural, and this makes for the best results on-screen.

Where can we find good ethical porn?

Ethical adult cinema is out there, but it is not free. In order to make it available and easy to access for those interested, I launched a new online cinema, Erotic Films (eroticfilms.com). It is a hub of ethical adult cinema where everyone can stream or rent my work, as well as the work of other brilliant ethical adult cinema directors. On this website, I curate films from a growing movement of directors who are trying to change the industry from within. I also host #eroticnights, where everyone is able to watch a film for free.

PART THREE

Doing It

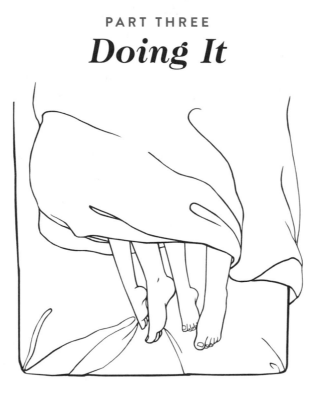

People always wonder what's normal—what they should be doing, and how often, etc. In our goal-oriented society, the truth that there is no normal is almost disappointing. It definitely seems simpler to check something off your list and move on, rather than go deeper and find out what you really like, what you wish for, and what you might not even have known you'd enjoy.

If we've learned anything from the experts here, it's that it's normal to get bored, and if you find yourself uninterested, it's also up to you to change it. Sometimes it's as simple as adding in some new options—and suddenly: interested. This part of the book is about making new options happen and potentially transforming old patterns that no longer serve you.

Once you know what you want and how to ask for it (see page 130), actually turning fantasies—whether it's next-level oral, adding a threesome, or trying BDSM—into reality takes some nerve, as well as lots of clear communication. Changing things up and trying different options might move you well past boredom—sex is, after all, supposed to be exciting.

CHAPTER 17

the antidote to bedroom boredom

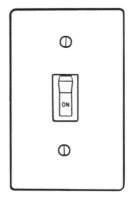

If you feel like you've lost the spark with your partner, be sure to check out psychotherapist Barry Michels's Q&A section (pages 51–59) on reigniting attraction. Also, for when we want to light a fire right under the bed, we have sexuality coach and Tantric expert Layla Martin on speed dial. While Martin assures her clients that it's normal to feel bored, and even uninterested from time to time, she also shows them (and us) that there are endless possibilities to explore so sex can stay fresh, exciting, and interesting—always. You just have to have the right tools.

Is It Normal to Be Bored?

LAYLA MARTIN

What does a healthy sex life look like?

A healthy sex life happens when both partners feel satisfied with the amount and quality of sex they are having. For each couple, this is totally different. One couple could be fully satisfied having one epic three-hour sex experience once a month, and that's healthy. Another couple could want sex daily, and that's healthy. It also depends on where you are at in your relationship—for a couple with kids, having deeply satisfying sex every other week could be a huge win. For a new couple, even a day apart may feel unhealthy!

What's unhealthy is when one partner's sexual needs are very unsatisfied—meaning they want to be having much more sex. Also, it's unhealthy if someone is having lots of sex they don't want to be having.

If two partners have unmatched drives, I work with them to find out how they can each compromise in a way that feels authentic to them. So the lower desire partner does what they can to feel more desire, to get in the mood, and to initiate sex more often; and the higher desire partner spends time either self-pleasuring or learning to be turned on without pressuring the other partner. It's important that they feel like partners on the journey to sexual fulfillment rather than adversaries.

Is it normal to feel bored with a longtime partner? Is feeling bored
*   cause for alarm?*

It's so normal to feel bored with a long-term partner. It's also totally normal to go through ups and downs in desire. To help couples understand this, I use the seasons as a metaphor: Each of us has a sexual desire season of spring, summer, fall, and winter. During your springtime, you can't get enough of each other; sex feels super exciting and there is a lot of flirting. In summer, you are incredibly passionate and turned on, and there's usually lots of sex happening. In fall, you let go of old habits and you may feel strange or off, like the chemistry isn't quite there. In winter, desire is usually very low, you lose interest in your partner, and there tends to be little sex happening.

If you understand your personal "seasons," and embrace them, then the cycle will keep happening and you will get back to spring and summer and sexual desire and play together. What happens, unfortunately, since so many of us have been taught only the fairy-tale version of sex, is that people in a relationship get into winter and then freak out. It can be scary to lose interest or get bored. And usually they don't talk about it—they don't work through it and the winter starts to last much longer than usual.

What helps a couple get back into spring? Intimacy exercises—talking, sharing, getting vulnerable with each other about hopes and fears. Spending erotic time together without necessarily having sex is huge. Too often in our culture we think sex is intercourse or nothing. But there are all of these amazing erotic practices you can do together when you aren't feeling that turned on to help move you back into attraction—like pussy and penis massage, sexual breath work, and eye gazing. This is one of the reasons I love a Tantric sexual practice for a couple—it helps them navigate the boredom of winter and get back into spring.

How do you know if your partner is bored?

It's different for every person, but generally your partner is bored if they aren't present with you during sex. If someone is fascinated, they show up. They are fully there. If they are bored, they start to check out.

How do you tell your partner that you're bored?

Don't tell your partner that you are bored. Tell them you want to explore. Tell them what you desire. Tell them you'd love to be sexually adventurous with them. Tell them you'd love to experience them in a new sexual way. Don't focus on the boredom. Focus on what you desire.

What do you find is the root cause of most of your clients' disinterest?

Most of the time, it's a lack of openness and vulnerability. I don't mean just sharing and talking, but cultivating deep intimacy. I find when a couple just talk, it doesn't necessarily lead to interest in sex. But when a couple go deep and they share their hopes, their fears, their deepest desires, and how they are really doing—the desire and great sex almost always come back. We aren't taught to be truly intimate in relationships; we're actually taught to hide our true selves out of fear. A lot of people stop showing their partner who they truly are, if they ever did in the first place. It's a kind of intimacy laziness and fear, and it leads to sexual disinterest.

Our cultural conditioning also creates disinterest. Many men are raised on pornography, and this trains them to be in their heads, and that leads to novelty seeking and a boredom with normal things. When you are out of your head and in your body—it feels scary at first, but it is inherently much more interesting.

I have also found that a lot of sexual trauma and fear of intimacy are underneath sexual disinterest. This is the main thing most couples don't understand about sex: When you are in a healthy, loving relationship, your sexual issues and fears come to the surface. No one tells us that—we just expect a fairy-tale. If you love the person, then sex should just work. Except it doesn't. If you really love someone, all of your childhood fears—of abandonment, of not being loved, of being trapped by commitment, or whatever it may be—start to come up.

When this happens most couples don't know what's going on, so they just shut down, which I find contributes massively to the lack of sex, and ultimately the experience of boredom in long-term relationships.

There is an epidemic of women who love their husbands and don't want to have sex with them, and this is a huge issue that no one is talking about. The answer to this epidemic is to make sex not just about pleasure, but also a forum for deep healing, for opening to the most vulnerable of intimacies, for total honesty, and for different emotions to flow. In this space, couples don't get bored sexually; they stay engaged because sex is more about personal development and creativity than pleasure.

There is an epidemic of women who love their husbands and don't want to have sex with them, and this is a huge issue that no one is talking about.

Boredom, though, can also just be people's laziness and lack of imagination. If your partner does the same thing again and again and isn't really present with you—that's bound to get boring!

What's the antidote to this boredom?

Tantric sex! In Tantra, you learn how to breathe and get wild and free, creative and spiritual. There is so much available to explore with one person, even for a lifetime, if you have the tools. The way to end boredom is to make sex not just about pleasure (or simply foreplay, intercourse, orgasm), but about a full range of emotional expression and experience, a full exploration of yourself and your partner. If sex is about healing, if it is about getting wild and primal, if it is about experiencing sacred states of gratitude and awe... it won't get boring.

One of the courses I teach to couples is a six-part exploration of the different types of sex—how to have sensational sex, electric sex, wild sex, Tantric sex, kinky sex, and enlightened sex—with various practices for each. For example: I like using breath work to induce trance states of ecstasy. Different massage techniques open up the body in profound ways. Very few women have fully explored their cervix or their full-body orgasm capacity, and very few men have explored their prostate and their multiorgasmic potential. Learning these tools and approaches makes sex surprising and continuously challenging and engaging.

Do you see any correlation between overscheduling sex and boredom, or is scheduling beneficial?

Scheduling is great—our modern lives are so busy and stressful that if we don't schedule sex, it's too easy to forget about it and go without. When I schedule sex with my boyfriend, even though sometimes it feels like a total drag, we are always so happy that we did, and it leads to even more natural sex.

Also, a lot of women aren't turned on by just the idea of sex. They need to actually be in a sexual situation to get turned on. So for women especially, scheduling sex can be really helpful because they won't get turned on until they are actually in a sexual situation. They might think they aren't attracted to their partner, but in reality, they just need to be naked and intimate with their partner to ignite their sexual turn-on.

The only downside to scheduling is that you can get lazy about seducing each other. You still want to remember that foreplay is happening all the time. Tease, flirt with, and erotically engage your partner throughout the day if you want the best sex. Don't wait until the scheduled sex date to turn it on.

CHAPTER 18

oral sex: giving vs. receiving

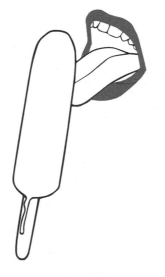

We've yet to meet someone who is neutral when it comes to oral sex. Whether you love giving or receiving, both, or could really do without one or the other, is largely a matter of personal preference—and to each her or his own, for sure.

But sometimes, oral is more complex: When it comes to receiving, it can be difficult to open yourself up in such a seemingly vulnerable way, even if you'd really like to—particularly if you're a serial giver in all aspects of your life, and/or if you're feeling self-conscious about the way your vulva looks or smells. On the flip side, there can be a lot of pressure to give the best oral ever—the internet is awash in step-by-step guides—which can take away what joy you might have found in going down on a partner. If any or all of this applies to you, you're normal.

If you'd like to feel more comfortable exploring oral sex, and certainly if you would like to feel more confident with your own body, keep reading for Juliet Allen's take on the psychology of oral and getting good at it. For more tips from Allen, a sexologist, sexuality coach, and kundalini Tantra practitioner based in Byron Bay, Australia, see her blog *Let's Talk About Sex* (noteworthy for the open-minded approach she takes to sexuality), where she hosts a podcast (*Authentic Sex with Juliet Allen*) and an online "Ecstatic Sex & Deep Intimacy" course.

The Psychology of Oral Sex

JULIET ALLEN

Can you talk about the psychology of receiving vs. giving?

When it comes to oral sex, most people often have a preference, whether they enjoy giving or receiving most. Like any preference, this can change and differ depending on who we are enjoying sex with.

When receiving oral sex, we are being invited to completely surrender to our partner and literally open ourselves physically and emotionally to pure pleasure. This can be a mind-blowing and breathtaking sexual experience that for some leads to intense orgasmic states.

For others, especially women, receiving oral is a really challenging experience. This is because receiving oral sex is all about surrender, and many women are afraid of surrendering to another person, and don't feel worthy of simply receiving pleasure and letting go. There are a lot of reasons for this: past trauma, a feeling of unworthiness, and body consciousness, to name a few. It's important to note that it's okay to feel this way, and that it's possible to work through this fear and gradually begin to open to the idea of receiving and surrendering to pleasure during oral sex.

When it comes to giving oral sex, most people are more comfortable with this because they either (a) feel like they "should"; or (b) love giving pleasure to their partner (and often feel turned on when they see their partner in sexual ecstasy).

When giving oral sex, though, lots of people focus on specific techniques rather than thinking of oral sex as an opportunity to worship their partner's pussy or cock. When we simply focus on oral techniques (e.g., licking her clit a certain way for a certain amount of time) we lose presence, and this can lead to dissatisfaction and disappointment.

> *When giving oral sex, though, lots of people focus on specific techniques rather than thinking of oral sex as an opportunity to worship their partner's pussy or cock.*

FROM THE GOOPASUTRA
BLOW JOBS

When we polled GOOP HQ about blow jobs, responses ranged from the practical—"Use both hands"—to an oddly insightful maxim: "The difference between a good blow job and great blow job is attitude." One staffer even shared something she learned from a (missed) BJ opportunity: "I had a lover who invited me one afternoon to come to his job to blow him in the broom closet. I declined, but as we discussed it by text message, I realized I was super turned on. I didn't expect that!"

What do you suggest to people who are self-conscious about receiving oral?

It's common for people, women in particular, to feel self-conscious about receiving oral because of body consciousness. I believe it's because women are often quick to judge the appearance, smell, and taste of their pussy. The best way to overcome this fear is to learn how to completely embrace the uniqueness of your own vulva and vagina. Get to know yourself intimately by looking at your pussy in a mirror, take time to massage her with love (I recommend using organic coconut oil), and be conscious about who you choose to allow inside you, energetically and physically. This goes for men also; embrace your penis for everything that it is and accept that it is perfect and worthy of love.

Another thing to consider is that people often feel like they earn love and acceptance by "giving" to their partner during sex. So people may find it hard to receive because it means they have to fully surrender to pleasure and receive love in a very intimate part of their body. If receiving during sex is challenging for you, I recommend exploring why that could be. When we get to know ourselves emotionally and sexually, we often find our experience of pleasure and orgasmic energy expands and evolves into something more fulfilling.

What about giving?

Let's be honest: Some people just don't enjoy giving oral sex, and that's completely okay. If that's you or your partner, then you may just have to accept that it's not going to feature highly in your sex life. Then again, some people don't enjoy giving oral sex because they don't feel confident in their oral skills. If that's you, I recommend exploring this and asking your partner what they enjoy and what they want.

How do you get good at it?

The key to getting good at oral sex is to authentically enjoy it. If you're enjoying it, your partner will sense that, and that's by far the biggest turn-on. Remember, your energy always speaks louder than your actions. In other words, suck his cock, or lick her pussy, with all your heart; moan, let your desire show.

The only other thing you can do is keep practicing—because practice makes perfect, right?—and tuning in to what your partner enjoys. It might also be helpful to attend sexuality workshops—there's always something to learn about all areas of sex, oral included. Other resources I recommend for learning more are books (like *The Art of Sexual Ecstasy* by Margot Anand and *Urban Tantra* by Barbara Carrellas); online courses (I have a free one available on my website); and connecting with a sexuality coach who will support you in living a sexually empowered life.

There can be a lot of pressure (on the giver and the receiver) for oral sex to end in orgasm—how do you approach this?

The biggest problem with all types of sex in our culture is that everyone is very focused on reaching the "end goal" of orgasm. Unfortunately, goal-driven sex, whether it be oral or penetrative, is problematic because it creates pressure for both partners to experience the often-elusive BIG O. Pressure to orgasm leads to anxiety, and most people end up spending a lot of time during sex thinking rather than feeling.

So, first, expand your definition of orgasm. Think of orgasm as waves of pleasure in your entire body, not just a mind-blowing explosion that marks the end of sex, but every single wave of pleasure you feel right from the beginning of sex. When you become more present and aware of the littlest of sensations, you are already experiencing orgasm. And remember, we all have orgasmic sexual energy naturally running through our body on a daily basis, it's just a matter of tapping into it and allowing it to flow freely.

How do you talk to a partner about wanting more oral sex?

The best way to talk about anything to do with sex is to be really honest and open with your partner. Sex is still such a taboo topic in the world, and, as a result, most people find it awkward to talk about what they want (*and* what they don't want). If you want to receive or give more oral sex, first tell your partner how much you love it, and then tell them how much you would love to experience more of it with them.

behind the blindfold

Is BDSM for You?

The BDSM spectrum encompasses a lot, from the fairly innocuous (you're wearing a blindfold) to the seemingly hard-core (you're in a dungeon). Maybe you already keep a feather in your toy box like Layla Martin (see page 40), but you are freaked out by the mention of a whip—or not. Whatever the case may be, there's much to explore in BDSM, and there's no one we trust more on the topic than Betony Vernon, author of *The Boudoir Bible: The Uninhibited Sex Guide for Today*. We first got to know Vernon for her jewelry designs meant to enhance sexual pleasure (e.g., a ring that doubles as a massage tool), and we were thoroughly impressed by her BDSM lair in Paris, which easily rivals Christian Grey's red room. Vernon tells us that the emphasis on pain in BDSM play is actually a misconception: Pain and pleasure being subjective, she argues that some might need more intense, direct sensation to feel pleasure, but that BDSM isn't meant to instill pain. How to do it right:

Getting Initiated into BDSM

BETONY VERNON

What is BDSM?

BDSM is the acronym for the matrix of bondage and discipline, dominance and submission, sadism and masochism. Those who seek the pleasures these ritualized sexual practices provide do not necessarily consider the genitals the primary focus of their sexual intentions. Lovers who enjoy BDSM play sometimes use the explicit, juxtaposed terms "master" and "servant" to describe the roles of the provider and the receiver of sensations. I prefer the words "top" and "bottom," respectively, to describe the activities that correspond to provision and reception of sensations. To bottom simply means to accept, and thereby submit to the sexual stimulation provided by their top. Likewise, one will top their bottom.

I encourage partners to explore the tools and techniques of full-body stimulation and to alternate between the roles of top and bottom in order to experience the mutual attainment of deeper levels of sexual satisfaction. After all, if we do not submit to pleasure, we cannot know its greater powers. Whether lovers categorize themselves as BDSM or not, great sex always plays with and stretches the lines between pleasure and pain. In its purest and most unleashed manifestations, the mutual attainment of deep degrees of satisfaction rarely has much to do with the sweet and tender illusions that Hollywood tends to propagate.

What BDSM behavior do you find people are most interested in exploring?

Over recent years, sexual practices that were once confined to the dungeon and considered by most to be the "dark" or "perverted" side of sex have gone mainstream. This includes erotic bondage (or restraint), which also happens to be one of the most common sexual fantasies. Erotic restraint, whether exercised with cords or cuffs, is a fun, sexy, and exciting way to explore the sexual realm together. When practiced skillfully between consenting lovers, it reveals unique sexual, emotional, and spiritual aspects of the partners. Erotic restraint does not benefit the bottom's satisfaction alone. The provision of pleasure is a great aphrodisiac; the pleasure of pleasing, combined with the effects of the power shift inherent to erotic restraint, imbues the top with a potent sense of sexual empowerment. The responsibility demanded of a top, who agrees to restrain his or her bottom, is also sustained by a surge of endorphins, which heightens concentration, overall awareness, and a sense of essential well-being.

Can bondage be for everyone? What do you need for a great bondage experience?

The positive outcome of any erotic bondage session hinges on consent, skills, and trust. Being aware of the ins and outs of erotic bondage allows lovers to avoid emergencies before they arise. Test out someone's receptivity to erotic motion restraint by simply telling them not to move; if this excites your lover, you can proceed to explore the art of bondage together. If, on the contrary, your lover freezes over, you may have to opt for other pleasures. Our sexual perception is deeply connected to our emotional and spiritual well-being, and not everyone should be expected to want to be bound.

Today, most lovers still consider great sex to be the ripe fruit of spontaneity and the idea of "planning" for sexual pleasure in advance synonymous with the extinction of the mysteries of sex.

How can someone bring BDSM into their sex life?

Today, most lovers still consider great sex to be the ripe fruit of spontaneity and the idea of "planning" for sexual pleasure in advance synonymous with the extinction of the mysteries of sex. Though it may be that good organization is irrelevant to the ephemeral outcome of "fast sex" and predominantly genitally oriented pleasures, forethought and good organization are as essential to the positive outcome of BDSM play as sexual skills and understanding. The pleasures of full-body stimulation are best provided through the use of tools, such as cuffs, cords, blindfolds, whips, floggers, and feathers. The effective use of such pleasure-inflicting instruments demands that lovers acquire the ability to use them to a safe and pleasure-maximizing end. Trust and consent, the foundation of all great sexual relationships, are as essential to BDSM play as good communication. Open and honest communication helps to maximize sexual pleasure by permitting lovers to get what they need to be fulfilled, to avoid the overstepping of each other's limits, and to prevent emergencies before they arise.

One of the most effective ways to initiate a lover to the possibility of exploring the tools and techniques of BDSM, and any ritual that entails full-body stimulation in a ritualized context, is to explore the powers of the seemingly innocuous blindfold. A blindfold that fits properly should shut out all light. Used with a trusted partner, a blindfold will give a clear indication of whether or not a lover will be open to exploring other forms of sensory restraint. Similarly, if your partner appreciates it when you spank them with your hand at the right time and on the right spot during erotic play, they probably will be open to exploring other forms of erotic flagellation.

Does BDSM always involve (some) pain?

This is one of the greatest misconceptions that surrounds BDSM play and is perpetuated by the media, cinema, and literature, among other sources. In reality, the perception of pleasure and pain is subjective. Some people simply need more intense and direct sensations in order to perceive pleasure, while other people may find that a feathery touch is more than enough to send them over the edge into sexual ecstasy. What one person may perceive as excruciating pain may be another person's greatest pleasure. Whether you are a full-blown masochist or vanilla to the core, if you perceive a sensation as painful, then your lover is clearly overstepping your limits. This needs to be communicated immediately, and if your partner persists, the session needs to be paused or come to an end. Establishing a safe word before the ritual commences is highly recommended.

exploring anal

W hile everyone seems to have an opinion when it comes to oral sex, there are arguably no topics in this book more charged than anal sex—something we saw firsthand in the amount and intensity of the responses we received to the first interview on anal sex that we ran on the site. That piece, with research psychoanalyst and author Paul Joannides, focused on media exaggerations of anal sex, the reality of it, and some safety concerns, including why condoms are so important (Joannides reported that HIV can be more readily contracted during anal sex); and why lube is a requirement (as it is painful without).

In his work as a sex and relationship therapist, Chris Donaghue, author of *Sex Outside the Lines*, addresses cultural phobias, hang-ups, and negative messages around sex—including anal sex. We interviewed Donaghue to further explore anal sex—both the act and how it's perceived.

The Charge of Anal Sex

CHRIS DONAGHUE, PHD

Why does anal sex seem to be such a lightning rod (no pun intended) in our society, and invite such extreme polarity?

Sex, in general, is always a highly charged topic, because even after much progression toward a more sex-positive culture, most people still have not found comfort and acceptance with their own sexuality or that of those around them. But anal sex—one of the most taboo topics—goes beyond this standard triggering, as it opens up a deeply entrenched cultural sex phobia and pushes the boundaries of heterosexuality and sex for fun and pleasure.

Traditionally, we are raised being taught that sex is for procreation, and always between a man and a woman. But anal sex rejects this, and is about sex for pleasure only, and not necessarily between a man and a woman.

Traditionally, we are raised being taught that sex is for procreation, and always between a man and a woman. But anal sex rejects this, and is about sex for pleasure only, and not necessarily between a man and a woman. Anal sex forces us to expand our safe and comfortable definitions of sexuality and also makes us encounter our bodies, especially our anal area, which is usually feared and ignored, and seen as dirty. Seeing anal sex as healthy and acceptable forces us to see our entire body differently, and to reconsider our sexual anatomy, along with messages about the purpose of sex (and heterosexuality) that may be ingrained.

How should you communicate with your partner about anal?

All sexual communication should be done confidently and honestly. Being sex-positive means proudly asking for the type of sex you want, using the correct terminology for your sexual anatomy, and never allowing a partner to shame you for being sexual or enjoying the type of sex you are aroused by. If a couple can communicate authentically about sexuality, then they have the skills to discuss all other important and triggering relational topics. This is why the health of a couple is demonstrated by their ability to talk about their sexuality. Anal sex carries a lot of shame—asking for it, prepping for it, and doing it—so use it as a way to work on relational communication and confidence.

What's in it for men? What's in it for women?

The anal area, anus, and rectum make up one of the most sensation-filled areas of the body, which is full of nerve endings and can be a big source of both pleasure and intimacy. The addition of a prostate gland for some, a thin wall between the anal canal and the vaginal canal for others (which can allow for indirect G-spot stimulation), and the universal presence of the perineal sponge for all, make for the potential for orgasm and fun.

One of the reasons some are turned off to trying or returning to anal sex is that many people aren't educated about it, and this can lead to discomfort and pain, or the continuation of body shame that ignores the anus as a potential site for pleasure.

FROM THE GOOPASUTRA
THOUGHTS ON ANAL

When we asked staffers for their thoughts on anal sex, we got the full spectrum of answers, ranging from never tried (but open)—"I'm not against it: I've been asked, but I haven't felt the urge to experiment with it. I keep saying that's something I'll try on a wedding anniversary..."—to, "Tried it. Didn't like it. The back entrance is exit only." And the affirmative: "Only option. Wonderful."

How can you prepare? What are other ways to explore the area?

Preparation for anal sex is not only a process of preparing for penetration and pleasure, it's also part of the process of developing the needed confidence and body relaxation. One of the flaws with anal sex for beginners is seeing prep time as only about hygiene and cleanliness. But getting ready for anal requires getting comfortable with your anal area because anal shame is one of the biggest blocks to enjoying this form of sex. Few people have taken the time to touch, look at, or play with their anus. Culturally, we see this area as dirty and useless except for its assumed purpose of the expulsion of feces. Not only is the anal area rich with pleasurable nerve endings, but it's also only a passageway for feces, not where it's stored, thereby making it far cleaner and penetration- and fun-ready than expected.

Prep for anal by talking about it openly prior to sex. Make it less taboo by discussing it with partners and friends. Many people these days are curious about trying anal sex, so it may be more welcome as a conversation topic than expected. Touch your anal area, look at it, play with it as often as possible. Get used to the experience of its being touched and associated with pleasure. Masturbate while stimulating your anus as well, to begin to eroticize this area, and associate it with orgasm and fun.

Nails should always be neat and manicured before playing with your or your partner's anus. You can start with toys—for example, small flexible dildos (use only ones made for the ass—meaning they have a flared base so as to avoid becoming stuck)—which helps train your anus for pleasure and insertion. Some men and women also prefer shaving or waxing their ass (yes, women, too) so as to feel cleaner.

What are the prerequisites of safe anal sex and common
    challenges?

Like all sex acts, the pleasure of anal sex is dependent upon arousal and relaxation. If you are stressed or anxious, your entire body will tense, including the anal area, which will not allow for ease or enjoyment of penetration. Practice, relaxation, and breathing are the three necessary anal sex prerequisites.

After that, the other obstacles are avoided by using lots of lube, slow insertion, and the use of additional penile or clitoral stimulation, depending on the anatomy of your partner. The anus and rectum are able to handle the insertion of a finger, toy, or penis safely, but the use of communication, lube, and slow initial movements are still needed as anal tissue is more delicate than vaginal or mouth tissue.

Enjoyable anal sex requires sharing what feels good or bad while being penetrated, asking your partner if it's arousing while penetrating them, and continually reapplying lube. Remember that the rectum is not a straight tube, and has curves and bends to it, so always try different positions to find the most comfortable, as everyone's body is different.

Does anal change a relationship?

Anal sex is capable of improving a relationship as pleasure and sex can be intimacy-building. Not all sex occurs to create bonding, but when it does, it's one of our most powerful and comprehensive forms of deepening relationship with another.

CHAPTER 21

asking for what you want

GP first turned us on to sex guru Laura Corn's book *101 Nights of Great Sex*, which comes with sealed envelopes containing instructions for seductions to try out on your partner. When you're deep into it with someone else, swapping sexual acts back and forth, the anticipation and the mystery of what suggestion the other will pull are hot in and of themselves. (If you're tech-inclined, there's also an app version of the book.) We reconnected with Corn, who is a big proponent of getting out of your comfort zone, for her take on how to know what you want and ask for it. Plus, we polled GOOP HQ to see the different ways staffers go about communicating desires to their partners.

Getting Out of Your Comfort Zone

LAURA CORN

How do we tap into our true wants and desires?

They say love is letting go of fear, but I think that also applies to great sex. If you're not tapping into your true sexual wants and desires, that means your insecurities or fears are somehow blocking you. (Otherwise, you would be going for it.) The best advice I can give is to tackle these fears one at a time.

First, write down your sexual desires—aim for at least five, perhaps as many as ten. Creating a list will help you come up with your game plan. Take those unfulfilled desires and rearrange them in an order from the easiest to achieve to the most challenging. For example, maybe you've always wanted to be blindfolded, spanked with a beautiful leather whip, or experience a threesome with another woman. Which seems the easiest to do? Start there and work your way down your list. It can be that simple—you'll become more confident with each step, and I guarantee that your sex life will get hotter and hotter. In the end, your fears will be a thing of the past.

What's the key to getting to know our own bodies better?

There's only one way to get to know your body better and that's through experimentation. Experimentation through self-pleasuring and trying new things with your partner (if you have one) are both important—and fun! It's a lifelong experiment of self-love, and what's exciting is that where you'll be in ten years will be completely different from where you are now.

Here's a quick story about how I learned to love my body: Up until my thirties, there was only one way I could have an orgasm, which was on my stomach. I would rock back and forth, grinding my hips into the bedsheets. I learned this technique at a very young age and never experimented with anything else. It did not serve me well. When I had sex with a partner, I was clueless, embarrassed, and fearful. I thought there was something wrong with me—I would never orgasm with a man inside me—and I couldn't reveal my *secret*, because that would be horrifying. This led to one failed relationship after another until I felt completely inadequate. I knew there must be a better way, and I desperately wanted to be in a healthy sexual relationship.

I eventually fell in love and wanted to be more sexually attuned with my body. I started reading books—a lot of sex how-to books (like *My Secret Garden*, *Women on Top*, *The Hite Report*, Kinsey Reports, and *The Joy of Sex*)—that opened up a whole new world to me. The more I read, the more comfortable and adventurous I became in bed. In the past twenty years, I've gone from being insecure to completely open-minded with my lover. Experimentation gave me the confidence to get to know my body better.

How do you tell a partner what you want?

Here are a few tips if you are having a hard time communicating what you want:

1. Watch an adult movie together. Point out what's hot and what's turning you on. If he or she isn't cluing in, go further, describing exactly what turns you on. But don't feel like you have to push anything on your partner, because I guarantee they are listening—and they might even surprise you beyond what you're imagining.
2. If you're a little shy, this one's for you. Simply highlight a passage from a sex advice book or an article that describes a fantasy you've always wanted to try. Have your partner read it while you two are in bed (watch them blush).
3. Want really steamy sex? Walk yourself into an adult novelty store. Choose that one (or maybe two, three, or four...) toy you've wanted to try but have always been a little intimated by. Gift wrap

them and give them to your partner over dinner (at a restaurant if you're feeling really bold) and watch their mind melt. You'll have fun that night. I promise.

What about during sex—how do you communicate without ruining the mood?

Communication should enhance the mood, not ruin it. It opens the mind to more possibilities. The more you exchange ideas, the more you stimulate sexuality. Each exchange only provokes and increases curiosity—and curiosity is the seed of passion.

> *Communication should enhance the mood, not ruin it. It opens the mind to more possibilities.*

On a more practical note, I think the tone of your voice is the key to connecting your desires to your partner's actions (just as it's important out of bed, too). Keep your voice gentle and loving.

Don't get too bogged down with giving tons of directions, though. A few sentences should be all it takes. Also, if your partner or you are not super verbal, a little physical helping hand doesn't hurt, either.

FROM THE GOOPASUTRA
ASKING FOR WHAT WE WANT IN BED

We polled the GOOP team, and their responses reflect the varying levels of confidence people have when it comes to speaking up for their desires:

- "Confidently and sensually. Unapologetically. Sometimes with show-and-tell; whatever gets the job done. In my experience, guys are enthusiastically responsive to direction, especially when it produces physical, audible results. Let's face it: Sexual prowess is at the core of the male ego. They're *psyched* to please. So if he wants to do it right, why not show him how?"

- "By literally asking."

- "I struggle with this. I'll wait until I can't take it anymore, and then I feel awkward bringing it up. I enjoy sex, but I feel nervous asking for what I want in the moment (or after), because I don't want the other person to feel that they're doing something wrong. Sometimes I have moments where I go for it and ask—if I'm comfortable with the person—and the verbal stimulation really turns me on."

- "If I'm in a relationship where I'm comfortable, I try to be vocal about it. If it's a new situation, I suck it up, or gently make suggestions in bed."

- "It took me some time to learn to do this. It became much easier once I was with someone I really cared about and trusted."

- "I straight-up tell them."

- "Very honestly. And particularly during sex."

- "Awkwardly make a joke out of it."

- "I think the best time is right after sex, when you're still lying in bed. You can kind of recap, saying, 'I liked that, do more of that'; or 'That wasn't working for me.' The information is fresh in your mind, but since the actual moment has passed, it takes some of the pressure off."

- "Moan more when something feels good. Go radio silent when something doesn't feel great."

- "I like to get started and see how things go. If I'm not being fully satisfied, I move his hand (or whatever we're using) to a better spot. If that doesn't work, I say what I want him to do."

- "I plant seeds that can blossom later. I'll ask for an expansion of the usual repertoire in a playful, encouraging way, but not in the heat of the moment."

- "Have an honest conversation about likes/dislikes, then experiment with other things from there. My boyfriend is more of the leader, so I follow along and then discuss afterward whether it was my cup of tea."

What benefit, if any, is there in going out of our comfort zone?

There's zero benefit in staying within your comfort zone. What are you learning? How are you keeping the spark alive? I certainly can't imagine a lifetime of comfortable sex without more variety, more foreplay, more surprises, more seduction.

Out of the thousands of couples I have spoken to, their biggest complaint is routine sex (i.e., missionary). Easy, but not *that* exciting. We all are hardwired to want something new, something fresh. Pure and simple novelty is the key to great sex.

Couples in long-term, fulfilling relationships consistently go outside their comfort zones. Whether it's doing something naughty in public, role-playing, or introducing your partner to a new toy—venturing outside the comfort zone is what elevates sex from the mundane to the magnificent.

But is it all about sex? No. Get out, do something new, have adventures. Ride a roller coaster, jump out of a plane together—just make some new memories.

playing out fantasy

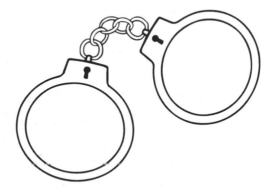

When we interviewed sexuality coach and Tantra expert Layla Martin about fantasy, we expected wild stories she'd heard over the years. In the past decade, Martin has spent some ten thousand hours teaching (primarily online courses), researching, and personally experimenting with sexuality. But in truth, Martin said that even when someone thinks they are the only person strange enough to have fantasy X, they're not alone—we all tend to fantasize about the same things. What does this mean? Martin breaks down what our fantasies say about us, how to accept and grow from the ones that might feel out of character, and, of course, her tips for playing out our deepest desires.

What Do Your Fantasies Say About You?

LAYLA MARTIN

What are some of the most common fantasies you hear about?

Being completely dominated by someone powerful, threesomes, getting lost in an orgy, desiring someone you're "not supposed to," and violent fantasies around aggression and danger.

Least common?

I actually can't think of "uncommon fantasies"—people tend to have similar fetishes, fantasies, kinks, and so on. Even when they think they are the only person in the world who could possibly fantasize about something that strange, it's my experience that they are not alone.

What's the difference between private and shared fantasies?

A private fantasy is something that's just for you. It feels erotic to have something that turns you on, and that feels like your little secret, as well as a space that is all yours. Especially in a long-term relationship, this kind of privacy can feel beautiful and important to a person. It helps to build a sense of erotic independence and agency (which is sexy itself).

I find that not sharing a fantasy is negative only when the person feels shame around it and not sharing is more like hiding it. Usually there is a sense that they'll be judged or rejected by their partner—and that kind of fear and shame isn't healthy for a relationship. If this is the case, it makes sense to first share it with a sex-positive therapist or coach to work on the feelings before sharing it with your partner.

A shared fantasy is something you share with a partner. Sometimes this is something you just talk about but continue to play out individually, and sometimes the two of you play it out together. In some cases, both people get turned on by the same fantasy, and then they share the turn-on of either talking about it or playing it out.

What do you think our fantasies tell us about ourselves and our relationships?

This is one area where I differ from a lot of the sex therapists and coaches out there. I have seen again and again in my work with clients that a fantasy isn't just a fantasy. It's a portal into what someone gets turned on by in the deepest parts of their mind—usually parts that are more unconscious or imprinted at a young age.

> *I have seen again and again in my work with clients that a fantasy isn't just a fantasy. It's a portal into what someone gets turned on by in the deepest parts of their mind—usually parts that are more unconscious or imprinted at a young age.*

Some of that is totally harmless—people get turned on by what they get turned on by. And in any case, fantasizing is totally fine—there is no reason to judge or shame it. But when someone starts doing deep sexual work and healing, their fantasies often transform.

Here's an example of how fantasies are reflections of early imprinting about sex: If you grew up in a patriarchal culture, your sexual fantasies can easily be a reflection of the patriarchy. Many powerful women find themselves fantasizing about being dominated against their will or treated poorly, and this isn't something they would want to experience in real life. I've spoken with women who have rape fantasies and they are horrified by this. Many men fantasize about treating women in ways they never would in real life.

I always work first to help clients embrace and accept their fantasies. Most of us started getting messages about sexuality at a very young age, and it isn't our fault if we carry imprinting that has us turned on by something that doesn't line up with who we are in the world or what we desire for our sex lives. It's okay to fantasize about something you wouldn't want to happen in real life.

However, I also work to bring consciousness and love into sexuality. A big part of having conscious self-pleasuring and sex is that it starts to feel more present and alive. It's the same as starting to meditate—you feel more present in life. What I've observed is that people who are highly disturbed by their fantasies see them evolve to reflect what they actually want when they bring consciousness into their self-pleasure and sex life.

Can you tell us what this might look like?

I used to be able to orgasm only when I had a fantasy about an older, powerful man having sex with a younger woman. This was a turn-on for a decade, but then it started to feel out of step with my own sexual empowerment journey and who I was becoming through my healing and Tantric practices. After I did several years of sexual transformation and deep Tantric practices, my fantasies transformed completely. I started fantasizing about sex where I was treated like a queen and was told beautiful, amazing things about my body and soul, and that became my deepest turn-on. It was pretty incredible. Finally, what I fantasized about matched up with what I truly desired. And I've seen this same process happen for many of my clients.

When we are sexually turned on and when we orgasm, we are actually in a highly creative, open, and impressionable state. What we think and feel impacts us deeply. So it makes sense to be aware of our fantasies and how they impact our experiences. If we're careful about what kinds of foods, emotions, and thoughts we have inside, why would we not ultimately want our sexual fantasies to be amazing reflections of our highest desires for ourselves and our sex lives?

Do you think fantasies can be a wedge between partners?

Fantasies can make you really un-present to your partner and your body. I recommend that people allow themselves to fantasize sometimes, especially when they are masturbating, but to also enjoy some sessions in which they focus only on the sensations in their body to keep them from being addicted to fantasy. After all, you feel so much more intimate and connected with your partner when you are both fully present together. To have that kind of sex, you want to train yourself to be able to get fully turned on and orgasmic as a result of being fully present to your body and your sensations and not just from fantasy.

How do you communicate your fantasy to your partner?

To create a safe container for partners to talk about their fantasies and desires, I have them do a communication exercise I call "Fears, Loves, and Desires": Ask your partner a question, and when they respond, only listen fully. Don't respond. Don't ask questions. Just listen and hold space for what they are sharing with you. Sit down across from your partner and ask each other these three questions (alternating, so you ask the first question, the partner answers, and then your partner asks you the first question, and so on):

1. What do you love about me?
2. What are you afraid of?
3. What do you desire?

This allows you to talk about your fears—of being judged, of being told "no," of being rejected, or whatever else you may be afraid of. Sharing desires and fantasies can be scary! This exercise also lets each partner talk about why they love the other. That means there is a foundation of love and appreciation set before you talk about your desires and fantasies. It will be much easier to hear and accept your partner after sharing fears and loves, which also opens you up and makes being honest easier.

Are there other things that will help if you want a partner to open up about their fantasies?

Take notice of what really seems to turn your partner on and ask them about it—if they would like more of it or to explore it more. You can ask questions like "If we could explore anything sexually together, what would you want it to be?" Or, direct: "If we were going to experience any fantasy of yours, what would you choose?" If you want your partner to share their true sexual fantasies, then you have to let them know that it is actually safe to do so. This means working to embrace your partner and accept their fantasies, as you would want them to do for you.

Do you have any tips for playing out fantasies?

When playing out a fantasy, it's important to get clear on what you both desire and want to experience. Discuss all the details and what each wants and what each is not willing to do. Be clear about your boundaries. Then plan it out together and decide how long it's going to last. You need to give your fantasy a good, clear container. That allows you to drop in and play it out fully, knowing that it will end. You can say something like "We're going to start the fantasy at 5 p.m. tonight and we'll do a closing process when it's done around 7 p.m."

After you play out the fantasy, it's equally important that you talk about it. How did you feel? What did you experience? What are you grateful for? This allows you to process anything uncomfortable or scary that could come up during the fantasy, and to digest the experience together, creating even more intimacy in the process.

FROM THE GOOPASUTRA
WHAT WE DAYDREAM ABOUT AT THE OFFICE
We asked GOOP staffers what they fantasize about when they're sitting at their cubicles, staring off into space...Here's

what they make of their daydreams (well, at least the ones they admitted to):

- "Most of my fantasies involve me in unrealistic lingerie hidden underneath a sexy black dress, followed by an intense sexual encounter with someone I can't have (read: my high school history teacher, an old coach, a certain friend's boyfriend). He rips my dress off and we have earth-shattering—yet tasteful—movie sex. Laughing as I write this: The sex is always tasteful."

- "Sex with much older men, like my friend's hot dad or a superior at an imaginary work environment."

- "Muscles. Strong shoulders. Being overpowered but still being in control. I don't feel like I have any uncommon fantasies."

- "I fantasize about being with a woman, even if it's just a one-time bucket list experience. I would be a pillow princess—the other woman services me, and I just enjoy. Or a threesome with another woman and a man."

- "Him being completely, utterly, overwhelmingly attracted to me and turned on. And wanting to please me in any way."

- "I think they're fairly common: being dominated, sex with a woman, having sex with someone I 'shouldn't,' sex with a stranger where it's 'just sex.'"

CHAPTER 23

sleeping around

Some would argue that there are never truly zero strings attached when it comes to sex. Maybe there's some truth to this: Doctor of human sexuality and relationship expert Emily Morse (who hosts the podcast *Sex with Emily*) says that it's difficult to totally remove emotions from sex (which is inherently charged), but that there are ways to keep things casual and satisfying if you aren't looking for commitment. What's more, there are pros to doing so, according to Morse. The irony of *casual* sex, though, is that it can get complicated despite the notion of effortless fun we might have had in mind. With her signature wit, Morse decodes the situation without sucking any joy out of it.

The Upside of Casual Sex and One-Night Stands

EMILY MORSE

How do you define casual sex?

Whenever we're talking about anything "casual," we think of a relaxed, temporary, or occasional situation. Meanwhile, sex is one of the most exciting, charged, emotional, and confusing subjects on the planet. It is the most intimate connection two people can share. So when you add the adjective "casual" to *sex*, things start to get tricky.

Sex is inherently emotional. When we try to remove our feelings, it's like eating dessert for dinner. It tastes delicious, and you fill up on it, but you still feel like you're missing something. However, it is possible for casual sex to be satisfying and empowering if you head into it with the right mind-set. Whether it's a potential one-night stand or a no-strings, friends-with-benefits situation, there can be plenty of upsides.

Casual sex is more accessible than ever, but this hasn't made it any less complicated. Even though the experience is supposed to be all about pleasure, if you regret decisions or feel emotions you didn't expect, your situation can become just as complex as any committed relationship. From the primal urge to procreate to the release of the "love hormone" oxytocin, we are hardwired to connect with each other.

What is casual sex then? It can be a precursor to love, a test-drive of a future relationship, or a period of self-discovery. It might be the result of an impulsive decision or of thoughtful planning. Casual sex is fluid, and for those who are able to go with the flow, it can be all of the above.

How do you know if you're ready for casual sex?

Deciding if casual sex is right for you starts with knowing yourself. If you're having sex to get back at your ex—you're not ready. If you're using Tinder to get as many matches as possible—you're not ready. If your self-esteem requires waking up in more strange beds than *The Bachelor*—you're just not ready. The point is if you imagine casual sex as a vehicle for revenge, as a solution to your problems, or as a way to artificially elevate your ego: You're. Not. Ready.

If none of that applies to you and your emotions are in check, a sexual connection without expectations or commitment may be something you're capable of. But even if that giant green light tells you to go for it, the truth is you won't know until you try.

How do you identify the right partner for casual sex?

When finding the right partner for casual sex, it's easiest to start with who you can rule out. No need to circle back to your ex—you already know that's a history of tangled emotions. Avoid your best friend's attractive sibling because even a positive experience could harm your friendship and strain their relationship. Your neighbors are always going to be, well, your neighbors, so when things don't work out, avoiding them will be a daily challenge.

So now, how do you find a casual candidate? The bottom line is that it all comes down to what you're looking for. Be honest about your intentions, and ask point blank if they can handle a casual situation. If they say they're typically a serial monogamist, it's best to keep looking. No one shows up at your door prequalified. The best thing you can do is to keep your eyes open, read between the lines, and trust your instincts.

How do you make sure you're on the same page as the other person?

I've got good news and bad news. The bad news is, even if you start off on the same page, the nature of your relationship is going to change. The good news is, all it takes is a little communication to get things back on track.

Even if you established clear intentions, it's very possible you'll wake up one morning and find that one thing you were originally turned on by now turns you off, or that your partner caught a serious case of the feels overnight. Change isn't just a possibility, it's pretty much guaranteed.

It's difficult to totally remove emotions from sex. I'm not saying it's impossible to keep things casual, just that the heart might be following a different plan than the brain. If things change unexpectedly, honest communication is the way to go. You're already having sex with this person—you'll survive a five-minute conversation, even if it's awkward. Open the conversation with something like "I really enjoy our time together, but I feel like things have been a little different lately—let's talk about it."

What's the key to having good casual sex?

One of the things that inspired me to start my podcast in 2005 was the fact that a lot of my friends were telling me they were having the greatest sex of their lives, but I wasn't sure I could say the same thing. I figured if sex was the most pleasurable experience on the planet, it would be worth it to really know what that meant—for me and for everyone.

Twelve years later, I can say with absolute certainty that there is not one answer (and it's not from lack of trying—buy me a glass of wine, and I'll tell you some stories). The point is, we should never stop learning. Here are a few of my favorite lessons:

Masturbating regularly is the best way to learn about your body. Take time to figure out what feels good and how you like to be touched. Once you discover what works for you, bring that experience to the party the next time you're with your partner.

Lose the pressure of having (or delivering) an orgasm. By some estimates, only about 30 percent of women orgasm during intercourse, and that stat is way lower in casual arrangements. Studies show that women are far more likely to reach orgasm when they feel an emotional connection with their partner—which isn't always the case when something is strictly casual. I'm not saying it's never going to happen, but if you take the focus off climaxing, you allow yourself to be present in the moment and enjoy all parts of sex. In fact, letting go and enjoying the ride will most likely lead you to that orgasmic place, anyway.

Casual sex is a great way to discover new things about yourself sexually, mentally, and even emotionally, especially if you have a healthy mindset and want to experience as much pleasure as possible. We tend to be a little less inhibited when we know the sex is temporary, so why not take the opportunity to set up your own sex ed curriculum? Tell each other things you've always wanted to try, explore new positions, and don't be afraid to ask for what you want. You'll soon recognize that the opportunities to learn and grow are endless.

We tend to be a little less inhibited when we know the sex is temporary, so why not take the opportunity to set up your own sex ed curriculum? Tell each other things you've always wanted to try, explore new positions, and don't be afraid to ask for what you want.

If the sex isn't great, should we work on it or walk away?

When I was a kid, if I complained to my mom that I was bored, she'd tell me, "Emily, only boring people get bored." I'm sure when she said that she never expected it to become sex advice, but here we are. (*Hi, Mom!*) The takeaway? If the sex in your casual arrangement is a little dull, before you blame your partner, realize that you're half of the equation. Casual sex is still sex; you get what you give. So if you're bored, chances are your partner is, too.

Now, I know you're thinking that the whole reason to go casual was to avoid the effort of a relationship. Sometimes great sex can be effortless—especially in the beginning. But when the newness starts wearing off, both of you may just start phoning it in. Here's where you're faced with the choice of making it better or making it stop.

If you're willing to do your part to bring back the heat, hopefully they'll reciprocate. If not, then your decision just got a whole lot easier.

How do you deal with the regret of a one-night stand gone bad?

If you find yourself with a bit of buyer's remorse over a casual hookup, take some comfort in the fact that you're not alone. A recent survey revealed that 81 percent of American women had one-night stands they didn't enjoy. Next-day emotions range from feelings of shame to fear and regret. Often, what we're feeling is more about how we see ourselves than anything the other person did or said. These moments of regret can be an excellent opportunity to learn about what we think we want vs. what we *really* want—or need.

The best thing to do is be kind to yourself. Be honest with how you're feeling and give yourself the time you need to process. Keep moving forward and do what you can to avoid a repeat of whatever emotion/issue is keeping you up at night.

Is there a difference between thinking of casual sex as a for-now thing or as a for-life thing?

For some, casual sex becomes a permanent way of life. I have friends and listeners who are perfectly happy balancing careers and their unattached sex lives. Some have incorporated casual sex into their marriages, either by opening up or swinging or having an occasional threesome. However, others have casual sex for a little while, and decide later on that they want a committed relationship. Then there are those who are constantly switching back and forth between casual and committed.

No matter where you fall on the casual sex spectrum, as long as you keep checking in with yourself, you're exactly where you need to be.

CHAPTER 24

adding a third

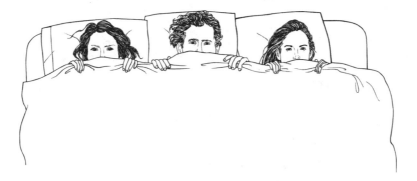

As with open relationships, regardless of personal preference, there seems to be endless curiosity around the topic of threesomes. Whether you'd ever entertain the possibility or consider it a turn-on (keep reading to see where GOOP staffers land here), Justin Lehmiller provides an interesting perspective on the question of whether or not to add a third to the mix.

Should You Do a Threesome?

JUSTIN LEHMILLER, PHD

When is it a good idea to have a threesome?
A threesome is worth considering only when it's something both you and your partner want—and you've taken the time to thoroughly discuss it

beforehand. It's not a good idea to jump into a threesome when one partner isn't fully on board or without first establishing some ground rules.

FROM THE GOOPASUTRA
MÉNAGE À TROIS

When we polled GOOP staffers about their threesome experiences, we got a lot of NAs, but we also got a range of responses about the threesome experience, which can be as varied in fantasy and actuality as any sexual experience:

- "I've had a few. My first one was with two complete strangers. I drank an entire bottle of wine to calm myself, but it turned out to be a lot of fun. I've had a few others with my SO, who was a virgin when we met. I brought up the idea that if he wanted to have sex with other people, then we should do it together."

- "I had a threesome with my then boyfriend and my (female) best friend. Overall, nothing to write home about—it was mostly fueled by curiosity."

- "In college, my best friend and I polished off a bottle of vino together, my boyfriend came over…and the rest is history. It wasn't as sexy as I'd envisioned."

- "No thank you. There are three things in life I never want to try… heroin, threesomes, and cottage cheese."

How can you make sure everyone has a fun time?

There are no guarantees that everyone will have a fun time, but there are some things you can do to increase the odds of a mutually satisfying experience. To that end, if you're thinking about having a threesome with your romantic partner—or, really, acting on any sexual fantasy with your partner—take the time to first identify all the potential pros and cons. Then talk about the areas of concern, make your boundaries clear, and come up with a mutually agreeable set of rules. For example, are there limits on which specific sex acts you'll do with the third person? What steps will you take to minimize potential health risks like STDs? How will you manage potential risks to the relationship, like one of you falling in love with the third? The goal here is to make sure you're both on the same page and comfortable with the arrangement of adding a third before anything happens.

> *At the same time, though, you both need to be realistic and recognize that no matter how much care and planning you put into a threesome, you won't know exactly how you'll feel until you're actually in that situation.*

At the same time, though, you both need to be realistic and recognize that no matter how much care and planning you put into a threesome, you won't know exactly how you'll feel until you're actually in that situation. For example, you might find it awkward at first, or maybe you'll feel unsure of what (or who) to do. Alternatively, you might find it distressing to see your partner getting turned on by another person—or maybe you'll find that it's super arousing! Basically, you have to be comfortable with a certain level of uncertainty and recognize that the situation might not be what you expect—it could be better or it could be worse.

What happens if the threesome becomes a twosome?

This is where setting rules comes in handy. Try to establish rules that will prevent a situation where one of you ends up unhappily sitting on the sidelines. Threesomes often become twosomes because one partner finds that they're just not as into it as they thought they would be, or because the third is really into only one of the partners. If either of these things happens, one of you will inevitably feel left out—and if you feel powerless to stop and exit the situation, this is the kind of thing that can end up causing a major fight and potentially destroying the relationship. So, to prevent this, you might want to establish a "safe word"—a word or phrase that will clue your partner in that the situation has moved beyond your comfort zone and you're ready to call it quits. The key here is to agree that either partner is authorized to invoke the safe word at any time, and to be perfectly clear about what it means: Effectively, one partner is revoking their consent, which means it's time to stop.

If it's a couple plus one, should the third person be someone you know or not?

There are pros and cons of each. For example, if the third is someone you know, odds are that you might have better communication with them and you might feel safer, too, both of which could end up improving the experience for everyone. Of course, if things don't go well, then you risk ruining that friendship. Also, because you're going to be seeing that person in the future, there are more opportunities for feelings to develop and for things to get complicated.

By contrast, if you don't really know the third and you're probably not going to see them again, there's likely to be less of an emotional risk to the relationship. At the same time, though, you're not going to have the same level of trust and communication, which might make for a less satisfying experience, and one in which the third might not be as respectful of your rules and boundaries.

As the third in a threesome with a couple, what should you consider?

Joining another couple for a threesome has the potential to be a great time for everyone, but it's important to recognize that you don't know exactly what you're getting into. It's possible that one partner is more into the idea of having a threesome (or having sex with you) than the other, which could make for an awkward situation. Also, if they've never experimented with group sex before, it's possible that one of them will feel jealous or uncomfortable once the action begins, perhaps because they didn't take the time to set up any ground rules at the start—so you might want to get to know the couple a bit before jumping into bed. Communicate and make sure everyone is on the same page; if it seems one partner is pressuring or coercing the other, that's not a good situation. Also, establish whether the couple has any specific rules or boundaries you should be aware of. Are certain sexual activities off-limits? If the couple seem to be inexperienced and appear not to have really thought things through, proceeding with a bit of caution isn't a bad idea.

In addition, be mindful of your own motives for joining this particular couple. Are you at least somewhat into both of them? Or are you really into only one of the partners and hoping that the threesome ultimately turns into a twosome? If it's the latter, there's a good chance this will turn into a scenario that no one really enjoys.

Have you found any similarities or differences based on gender or sexual orientation when it comes to threesomes?

In the research I've conducted, I've found that threesomes are one of the most popular sex acts people fantasize about, regardless of their gender and sexual orientation. In other words, most—but not all—people have fantasized about a threesome before. However, when it comes to the prospect of taking part in a real-life threesome, men tend to be more interested in it overall than women—and that's true regardless of sexual orientation.

Why is that?

At least among heterosexual adults, men and women seem to think about the prospect of a threesome quite differently. Men are more likely to anticipate pleasure and fulfillment, whereas women are more likely to anticipate that they would feel used and that they would be harmed. It's this difference in expectation that contributes to women's lower interest in having a threesome.

One other gender difference that emerged in my research is that, among heterosexuals, men are more interested than women when it comes to threesomes involving one male and two female partners. However, women are more interested than men when it comes to threesomes involving two males and one female; straight women are also more interested than straight men when it comes to having three-somes with only persons of the same gender, something that may be due to the fact that women tend to be more sexually fluid than men. Therefore, generalizing, we do see some differences in the kinds of threesomes men and women are open to having.

PART FOUR

Orgasm

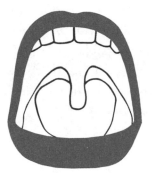

It used to be that women weren't really supposed to enjoy sex so much—which is no good—and they certainly weren't expected to orgasm. Today, despite a more evolved perspective and significantly more sex education, we still get the same amount of information on pleasure we used to (zero). At the same time, there's now more pressure on both men and women to orgasm: On our phones and laptops, there's a secondary "education" system full of performances of women achieving orgasm—through a method that may work for only approximately 5 percent of the female population.

So the pressure is on to have an orgasm, on schedule, in a particular way that doesn't work for most women. Or simply perform it.

Our aim here is to stop the performance and have the experience. Most of us orgasm when we masturbate, so start with more of that (particularly because, as Alexandra Jamieson observes, the culture is full of acknowledgments of male masturbation, while the female equivalent remains taboo). Who are you when no one is watching—and how can you bring that person, and what excites her sexually, to your relationship?

When we expand our definition of orgasm, a new world—one without a script, or at least less of one—of possible pleasure starts opening up. There's no goal, no predetermined pace, no box to check, just our actual selves, our experiences in the moment, and imagination, creativity, and pleasure.

CHAPTER 25

orgasm equality

I ntercourse" is regularly used interchangeably with "sex"—we're guilty of doing it (pun!) as shorthand—and yet intercourse is not equivalent with sex, and certainly not the only activity at the party. While there's nothing wrong with penetration, the hype it gets is disproportional considering that most women—as many as 95 percent, says sex therapist/psychology professor Laurie Mintz—achieve orgasm from clitoral stimulation. As Mintz puts it: Many of us are so focused on doing what we consider fucking (i.e., intercourse) and not on enough other sexual activities that it's resulted in a major pleasure gap. The stats, gathered from her clients, college students, and research on how often women orgasm vs. men (for her appropriately titled book, *Becoming Cliterate*), sting. We asked her how we can remedy this to benefit women—and men.

Becoming Cliterate

LAURIE MINTZ, PHD

What are the main stats around the pleasure gap?

There are many studies on the pleasure gap between women and men (too many to list); the most striking I've come across are the following:

- In one survey of thousands of women and men, 64 percent of women vs. 91 percent of men said they'd had an orgasm during their most recent sexual encounter.
- Another large-scale survey of university students found that 91 percent of males and 39 percent of females report always or usually experiencing an orgasm with a partner.
- In a survey of over 2,000 straight women, 57 percent said they orgasm most or every time they have sex with a partner, while 95 percent said their partner orgasms most or every time.
- Finally, in anonymous surveys I conduct with my own students (across about four years and over 500 students), 55 percent of men vs. 4 percent of women said they usually reach orgasm during first-time hookup sex.

How does the pleasure gap vary across generations and between committed vs. noncommitted relationships?

I don't know of any study that actually compares the pleasure gap by age—but here is a related finding: Research shows that women's frequency of orgasm and sexual satisfaction increases with age. As women age, they generally get more comfortable with themselves and are more able to say what they need sexually. But as I tell young adult women, there's no reason to wait to get older to become orgasmic and satisfied. A woman of any age can get to know her own body, feel entitled to pleasure, and learn the skills to tell a partner what she needs during sex.

With respect to how the gap varies across relationship contexts—that answer is clear. The orgasm gap is widest between the sexes during first-time hookup sex, but progressively narrows with subsequent hookup sex, friends-with-benefits sex, and relationship sex. But it never closes altogether, even in relationship sex.

FROM THE GOOPASUTRA
THE WATER-GLASS ANALOGY FROM
THE BRILLIANT PEGGY ORENSTEIN

Peggy Orenstein, author of many books, including the recent bestseller *Girls & Sex*, brings up an important pleasure-gap-related point. She was talking with us about lack of reciprocity in oral sex (and her related research), but her apt metaphor applies to sexual interactions across the board:

"Sometimes I'd ask the girls I interviewed: What if every time you were with a guy, he told you to get him a glass of water from the kitchen, but he never offered to get you one? Or if he did, it was totally begrudging, like, *[big sigh]* 'You want me to, um, get you a...glass of water?'

"You would never stand for it! So why do you consider it less insulting to be repeatedly asked to give a blow job without reciprocation than to be asked to get a glass of water from the kitchen?"

What's behind the pleasure gap?

The number one reason behind the pleasure gap is that we are doing too much of what we consider "fucking" (aka intercourse) and not

The number one reason behind the pleasure gap is that we are doing too much of what we consider "fucking" (aka intercourse) and not enough of other sexual activities.

enough of other sexual activities. We overvalue men's most common way of reaching an orgasm (intercourse) and undervalue women's most common way (clitoral stimulation). Despite media and porn images of women having fast and fabulous orgasms from penetration, it's estimated that only about 5 percent of women are able to orgasm from penetration alone. The other 95 percent need some form of clitoral/vulva stimulation—either alone or coupled with penetration.

Here are a few other reasons:

- We have a double standard that judges women more harshly than men for having casual sex. This leaves many women feeling conflicted about the sex they're engaging in. It's hard to have an orgasm when you're guilt-ridden.
- We're bombarded with media images of "sexy" women whose role is to attract and please men. These images are plentiful in porn, but they're not limited to porn—open any magazine and you'll find advertisements using gorgeous, provocatively posed, scantily clad women to sell everything from cars to clothes. Researchers have found that these images lead girls and women to constantly assess how they appear to others. This puts women's main focus on being sexually desirable to others rather than on their own sexual desires. It places women's emphasis on how they look rather than on how they feel. Even worse, some women (and men) come to believe— even subconsciously—that a woman's main role is to please men, rather than believing sex entails equally giving and receiving pleasure. A logical consequence of this is that some women gauge how good a sexual encounter is by their partner's pleasure rather than their own (i.e., "If it was good for him, it was good for me").

- These same media images of sexy, beautiful—and thin—women are also the main culprit in the fact that many women dislike their own bodies. And a woman who dislikes her own naked body is not going to feel open and free during a sexual encounter. It's impossible to have an orgasm while trying to hold your stomach in (believe me, I spent my younger years trying).
- Sex education focuses almost exclusively on the dangers of sex, such as pregnancy and sexually transmitted infections (STIs). Stating the obvious, you're less likely to enjoy something that's been billed as perilous rather than pleasurable.
- Most women (and men) have zero training in sexual communication. Good communication is especially necessary when it comes to female orgasms. Most men pretty much reach orgasm the same way and it's not all that complex. It's a lot more complicated for women to orgasm, since there are vast differences between women in terms of what they need to orgasm. Also, what a woman needs can vary from one encounter to another. Men can't read minds—or vaginas. Sexual communication is needed for women's orgasms, yet it's a skill rarely taught in sex education.

Where'd we go wrong?

Women's sexuality and orgasms have a long history of being negated, starting all the way back with the Greeks and the Romans. There was a brief period of time (the 1960s and 1970s) when women were learning about and talking about their clitorises, but we've never overturned centuries of belief about the supremacy of intercourse. In terms of modern history, I peg a lot of the problems on Freud. Despite knowing that the clitoris was central to female orgasms, he started the big lie (i.e., that women should orgasm from intercourse alone) we're still struggling with today. In Freud's own words, he said that once girls hit puberty, "the clitoris should...hand over its sensitivity, and...its importance, to the vagina." In essence saying: Grown women who need clitoral stimulation to reach orgasm are defective.

Worsening the problem has been all the media hype about the "G-spot." In 1982, three scientists wrote a book, titled *The G-Spot*, about an area in the vagina that, when stimulated, can lead to orgasm in some women. They also wrote about female ejaculation. The authors of *The G-Spot* provided evidence of different types of female orgasms—clitoral, vaginal, or a combination of the two called a "blended orgasm"—while also emphasizing that there is no one right way for a woman to orgasm. However, the message picked up by the media was that if you aren't having G-spot orgasms with accompanying female ejaculation, you are seriously missing out. G-spot orgasms became big business (e.g., in the forms of books, movies, and sex toys to help find it). Beverly Whipple, one of the scientists who wrote the original book, has tried to remind the public that she never wanted G-spot orgasms to be a goal to achieve. But her voice seems to have been lost. Some feminists say that this hype about the G-spot has set us back to a Freudian era of women searching in vain for vaginal orgasms—leaving them feeling inadequate and unsatisfied.

What role did clitoral stimulation play, evolutionarily speaking?

More than twenty evolutionary theories have been proposed (though none proven) on the adaptive value of female orgasms. Some theories focus on how orgasms help a woman to feel bonded with her partner, and others focus on how orgasms promote conception.

One theorist, Elisabeth Lloyd, wrote a book debunking all these theories, and positing her own theory (which also hasn't been proven), that the female orgasm serves no purpose at all and is just a fantastic bonus of fetal development. She pointed out a faulty assumption underlying all theories about orgasm and conception: If an orgasm were needed for conception, most women wouldn't conceive since they don't orgasm during intercourse.

An exciting, newer theory proposes the past function of female orgasm. Two scientists (Mihaela Pavlicev and Günter Wagner) discovered that some other female mammals release the same hormones (oxytocin and prolactin) during mating that female humans release during orgasm—and that in these other species, eggs are released only during mating. The discovery led Pavlicev and Wagner to speculate that the clitoris used to be located inside the vagina—causing our ancestors to orgasm during intercourse in order to send hormonal signals to the brain to release an egg. This worked well when we rarely encountered males, as it helped us to make the most out of each mating encounter. But when mating started occurring more regularly (due to our ancestors' spending more time in social groups), it was no longer adaptive to release an egg each time one mated. Eventually, our female ancestors evolved a new system of releasing eggs in a regular, monthly cycle instead of each time they had intercourse. And, so as not to confuse the old and the new signals for ovulation, the clitoris moved away from its original position inside the vagina.

Another theory (my all-time favorite) proposes that women's *inability* to orgasm during intercourse is adaptive because it helps women pick out mates who will be attentive to their needs. In other words, a mate who is concerned about his female partner's clitoral-based sexual pleasure is going to be a good mate overall.

> *Another theory (my all-time favorite) proposes that women's inability to orgasm during intercourse is adaptive because it helps women pick out mates who will be attentive to their needs.*

How can women in hetero relationships feel more pleasure from sex?

The formula is simple—although it's not that simple to implement due to our cultural scripts about how sex should go (i.e., foreplay to get her ready for intercourse, intercourse, male orgasm, sex over). Here's the formula:

- Pleasure yourself so you know what you need to orgasm.
- Feel entitled to get that same pleasure and orgasm during sex with a partner.
- Use good sexual communication skills to tell your partner what you need to orgasm, and/or touch yourself during partnered sex (i.e., rub your clit during intercourse).

The most essential step to orgasming with a partner is getting the same kind of stimulation you get when pleasuring yourself. When women pleasure themselves, 94 percent reach orgasm. Women generally know what to do when they are alone, but when having sex with a man, they relegate this type of stimulation to second place or expect to orgasm from a different kind of stimulation (e.g., penetration).

Some women prefer to receive clitoral stimulation without penetration (e.g., oral sex or manual stimulation), while others prefer to pair clitoral stimulation with penetration. She or a partner can use a hand or a vibrator. Many (but not all) women who use this method say they prefer to "do it themselves," since they best know what they need at any given moment. There are also wearable vibrators that provide clitoral stimulation during intercourse (e.g., a cock ring with a vibrating clitoral extension attached).

Anything (else) in particular that male partners in hetero relationships should know?

They should learn about female genital anatomy—and about how the vast majority (or even all) of the nerve endings that most women need to orgasm are on the outside, not the inside. Since what every woman needs to reach orgasm differs and can differ even from one time to another, they should ask a woman what she wants or needs (e.g., "Tell me how to pleasure you"). Men should also be ready to take their time—the average woman needs twenty minutes of clitoral stimulation to orgasm. Similarly, they should spend more time in warm-up (e.g., kissing, touching other body parts, caressing all over) before heading to the genital region—I recommend fifteen to twenty minutes. Finally, they should know that being cliterate—or knowing about women's pleasure and orgasm—benefits them, taking the pressure off them to thrust hard and last long to "give" a woman an orgasm.

What should we be doing differently on a societal level?

Our sex education system is sorely lacking when it comes to pleasure in general and female pleasure in specific. Only twenty-three states in the United States mandate sex education, and only thirteen require medical accuracy for the programs. Most sex education in the US is about the risks of sex (e.g., unwanted pregnancy, sexually transmitted infections) and fails to mention sexual pleasure. Even the most progressive sex education classes cover only women's internal anatomy. As stated by Peggy Orenstein (author of *Girls & Sex*) when describing US sex education, it's "as if the vulva and the labia, let alone the clitoris, don't exist."

Our cultural language also mirrors—and exacerbates—this problem: We use the words "sex" and "intercourse" as if they were one and the same; we hesitate to say the word "clitoris," and instead, we call all of women's genital anatomy a "vagina"—the part that's sexually more useful to men.

Finally, just watch almost any movie with a sex scene. To quote one of my male students, "In the porn I watch, it's male pounding that turns women on." To quote one of my female students, "In mainstream movies and in porn, all I see are women having orgasms during intercourse." It's no surprise that the most frequent question asked by my female human sexuality students is: "How do I have an orgasm during intercourse?" Women's magazines often answer this question by recommending specific intercourse positions, which makes matters worse, because it implies that all women will orgasm during intercourse if only they do it right.

Do you think that any porn can have a positive effect?

There is some porn, categorized as "feminist porn," that often gives more realistic models of female pleasure and orgasm. Many women enjoy watching porn for its arousing, erotic effects. Women are, like men, very visually aroused, and there's evidence that women are aroused by all kinds of porn (e.g., heterosexual women are aroused by lesbian porn and vice versa). Interestingly, one study showed that women who watched porn in which women touched their clitorises during intercourse were more likely to model this behavior. Still, in watching porn, people need to keep in mind that it is for entertainment and staged, so it's not often realistic.

CHAPTER 26

is the g-spot a real place?

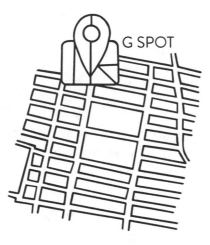

Psychologist and neuroscience researcher Nicole Prause (who founded the sex biotech company Liberos) looks at what's happening in the brain when we're engaging in a sexual experience. Some of her work confirms what we intuitively "know" about sex, but a lot of it overturns long-held beliefs. Here, science weighs in once and for all on the G-spot (stop searching for it); female ejaculation (if you don't, who cares?); masturbation (truly not wrecking relationships); and more myths.

Busting Sex Myths

NICOLE PRAUSE, PHD

Is the G-spot a real place?

If you put your fingers inside your vagina, the anterior vaginal wall is toward your belly (not your back, butt, or sides). There is no spot on the anterior vaginal wall that has a unique anatomy or is consistently placed across women, so there isn't a standard for finding areas of sensitivity. The nerve density of the wall isn't consistent—if you sample from different places across the wall in different women, the number of sensitive receptors will vary. Women also report that this sensitivity varies with their menstrual cycle, so sensitivity on one day may not be present a few days later in the same woman. There is no known harm in stimulating these areas. I would treat stimulation of the anterior vaginal wall like any new sex toy—a fun curiosity that might provide extra pleasure in your sex life.

What about female ejaculation?

Many women report the sensation of expelling liquid during sexual arousal, sometimes with orgasm and sometimes not. There isn't a thorough survey to tell us what proportion of women experience this, but it is well documented in the laboratory. Studies show that the liquid is urea from the bladder (possibly with minute amounts of lubrication mixed in from collection procedures). There aren't any documented benefits of female "ejaculation."

How does being in an aroused state differ from experiencing an orgasm?

High sexual arousal does not look very different from orgasm. Scientists long assumed orgasm had special rewarding properties, but I now question whether this is true or if orgasm just involves a little more of the same changes we see with high sexual arousal states. However, the very early stages of sexual arousal seem very different from later stages. Early on in sexual fantasy, viewing sex films, and even starting to masturbate, the brain has evidence of effort. This could mean that we need to reach some level of sexual arousal to be able to start to try to orgasm, but then the brain must "let go" from a neuro-control perspective to start to try to experience orgasm. If anything, orgasm itself seems to bring us back around to conscious, aware states.

What have you found to be untrue about sex that contradicts most people's beliefs?

People assume masturbation harms romantic relationships, whether from social isolation, biologically imprinting nonintercourse stimulation, or creating misogyny when done with adult films. But masturbation has overwhelmingly positive effects on health, from boosting mood to acting as a sleep aid (somnolence) and balancing discrepant desires in a relationship. Further, the idea that we "shouldn't have to" touch ourselves during partnered sex may prohibit our partner from learning what pleasures us, or serve to stigmatize and shame a common practice.

What test results have most surprised you at your lab?

We tested some women who claimed to be multiply orgasmic. We found that they actually were not having the contractions scientists expect to see to verify the presence of orgasm. This raises the very real possibility that women who report atypical, high-frequency orgasm patterns might be talking about a completely

Yet another reason why women should not aspire to try to replicate what they read in magazines: Who knows if the writer has any insight into what their body is actually doing!

different experience. Yet another reason why women should not aspire to try to replicate what they read in magazines: Who knows if the writer has any insight into what their body is actually doing!

FROM THE GOOPASUTRA
THE FEMALE SATISFACTION SURVEY

We regularly get inspiration from readers, whose curiosity is at the heart of this book—which is why we decided to reverse roles and ask *them* some questions: *Are they satisfied with their lives? Their relationships? The sex they're having?*

Of the 1,700 women (and handful of men) who responded, more than three quarters were in a relationship or married, and about half had kids, and almost 80 percent worked outside of the home. The majority were satisfied with their careers, relationships with their children, and their partners.

Sex, though, was a different story: Only 37 percent were wholly satisfied with the quality of their sex life, plus: 72 percent felt like they should be having more sex (about half believed they have sex less frequently than their peers) and 67 percent wished they orgasmed more.

For us, this survey was another reminder the intimate slice of life is the hardest one to get right for many of us—or, at the very least, there's room and good reason to seek improvement.

---

orgasmic meditation

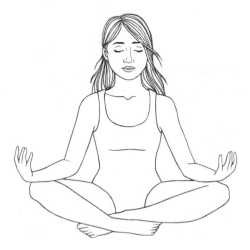

If you have the opportunity to hear Nicole Daedone speak, take it. Daedone, who is known as the creator of Orgasmic Meditation (OM), can be found these days alternating between New York City (where she is writing her next series of books and building a media company based on the lifestyle of OM) and at The Land, an idyllic sanctuary in the wilderness of Northern California which hosts a variety of retreats designed to truly recharge the battery. Just being in Daedone's presence is like an electric shock to the system (in the best way). A lot of sex talk puts you in your head, but Daedone puts you in your body—and makes you want to *do*.

OM, the practice that is central to Daedone's work, is essentially the yoga of sex, whereby a woman lies down and her partner strokes her clitoris for fifteen minutes, and both reap the benefits (enhanced connection, happiness, vitality, and fulfillment) of tapping into a higher orgasm state. Here, Daedone makes the persuasive case for trying OM, for letting your desire lead, and for orgasm taking over the world (we're ready).

The Future of Pleasure

NICOLE DAEDONE

What is the practice of Orgasmic Meditation all about?

It's a practice that combines the power and attention of meditation with the deeply human, deeply felt, and connected experience of orgasm. When I first tried OM, I had a life-changing experience. It was so profound, so "Oh! This is what is supposed to be!" that I began to investigate the question: What would happen if we rebuilt the erotic from the ground up, but this time included consciousness and spirituality? In the same way that we have been moving from processed to whole foods, from mere fitness to yoga, OM shifted sex out of the dark, from under the covers, from the shameful and often consumptive places where it used to be, and into the light. Here we can have experiences that foster our well-being. We take the most powerful impulse, the sex impulse, and approach it in an entirely new way. OM offers a practice through which we can harness this impulse that is a deliberate, repeatable method for accessing orgasm.

There's a distinction that's worth making: I differentiate between climax and the orgasm state. Climax is a few seconds of physical experience, whereas the state of orgasm is continuous—more akin to an optimal state of consciousness brought about from the activation of the erotic impulse. It's the feeling of being so completely absorbed in an experience that there is no psychic chatter, no being "stuck in your head"; it's a falling-away of the ego. When this happens, our sense of limitations falls away as well. In the orgasm state, we feel totally present and connected, as if a deeper intuitive sense has awakened—and this has cumulative positive effects that carry over into everyday life.

Much of OM is about tapping into the sensitivity and sensation of the clitoris—how?

There are roughly eight thousand nerve endings in the clitoris, and as you begin stroking, those nerve endings become sensitized. The most sensitive spot is the upper left-hand quadrant of the clitoris, the "one o'clock spot." If you've ever said (or thought): "No, a little to the left; no, a little to the right," you're trying to get your partner to the spot. When the spot begins to open, what happens is, as sensitive as that one very, very elusive spot is, the entire clitoris gets to be. As you stroke more, over time (say after a year), your entire genitals become that sensitive. As you stroke even more, the entire body gets turned on, and you're restored to your birthright of a turned-on body—one that can feel all the sensations available to it.

Why are so many women conflicted about orgasm?

I've worked with tens of thousands of women, and I've not once seen a woman who couldn't access the orgasm state. I've met women who can't climax in the way a man does, but I've never seen a woman who isn't capable of entering the state I'm talking about.

Women are conflicted because the options available to them are not the options that suit their bodies! They're based almost entirely on a confining definition of climax. For instance, reading arousal in a woman's body is often more challenging than in a man's. We're conditioned to think "orgasm" can be present only when there's a huge peak and release of energy (with all the attendant thrashing and moaning). But arousal can be so much subtler. You can tune in to it through swelling, wetness, contractions of the vaginal walls, pulsing, buzzing, tingling, and many other sensations. Many people have these experiences but discount them, because they don't conform to the conventional definition we have of orgasm.

Not only that, but women also contend with a much higher vigilance center—the part of the mind that's always on the lookout for threat or danger. To get our minds to relax, root into our bodies and simply feel, is generally a more challenging task for women than for men. We're thinking about picking up the kids, the meeting at work tomorrow, how our bodies look, and on and on. So to have a practice that allows a woman to soften and shift her attention to how she actually feels is invaluable. It's like she gets a temporary reprieve, to totally relax, and to come back refreshed and with a whole new perspective.

So are we predisposed to feel conflicted about pleasure—is this different for men and women?

I think it's different for women and men on the surface but it is fundamentally the same challenge. It's as if men and women are going through different labyrinths to get to the same place in the world. The caveman brain that we (all) have is oriented toward the negativity bias, toward always looking for the problem. We look to shrink reality to fit an idea, and then we look to stabilize everything and make it permanent—and that's not how reality is. It's impermanent. For me, pleasure isn't some kind of *ah, bliss* state. It's the capacity to be with things as they are. When I can do that, nothing could be more beautiful.

How do we get to that place of deep pleasure?

Let your desire lead. As women, we are often taught that our desire is indulgent or selfish, but true desire is at the foundation of all great things—from relationships to innovation. It's the only force powerful enough to pull us out of the everyday routine of life, or the muck and mire we sometimes get stuck in. I've always noticed that beneath every complaint is actually a desire, so we train people to go straight for speaking the desire—for example, instructing your partner on what pressure, speed, and intensity you want in a given moment.

To get in touch with your desire, focus on what you do feel instead of what you don't—and start with the present: "From here, this is what I want." Desire doesn't think in hypotheticals. It doesn't start with a fantasy of the future that's subject to change, nor does it start with what isn't enough. It begins here and now, with the countless circumstances it's attuned to. Living from your desire requires you to acknowledge what's going well and be grateful for all the good in your life. From this state, you recognize how rich and abundant your life is already: that you have everything you want, that there is room for more. You are not coming from a place of need or desperation, which would compromise your ability to pursue what you want. When we come from a place of overflow, we have the capacity to give without losing ourselves and to receive without cheapening the gifts we've been given.

If you're struggling to get there, start with your body. Remember that it knows what you want. Listen to the hungers that whisper and the ones that roar. Pay attention to the magnetic fields that draw you toward one person and away from another. Ask out that person you've been afraid to talk to. Book that trip you've been depriving yourself of for no good reason. Give your thinking mind a vacation and let your orgasm make your decisions for a day. (Or a month.) Live in your turn-on. Say yes when you want to say yes. Say no when you want to say no. If you don't know, say maybe, but don't give in. Follow your desires without dumbing them down. They may not lead where you thought you wanted to go, but they will never lead you astray.

Where do you think monogamy fits into following your desire and feeling fulfilled?

Right now, we have this model of monogamy, and it's as if the map doesn't match the territory—it doesn't actually get you where you want to go; it doesn't deliver on its promise. The paradigm of monogamy needs to be shifted so that it allows for our lives to get better the longer we are in a monogamous relationship. Similar to Maslow's hierarchy of needs to reach higher consciousness, a monogamous relationship has to hit five triggers to really be fulfilling: (1) You have to feel safe; (2) you have to feel that you're choosing to be in this experience; (3) you have to feel connected to the person; (4) you have to feel like you have variety; and (5) you have to feel growth. Often, the way we try to satisfy those needs is dysfunctional: For instance, many people seek variety by having an affair. We don't actually learn to have nuance with our partner. Or, the way we learn to have growth is that we actually consume more. We get more, rather than learning how to find deeper patterns of connection and intimacy with each other.

If we can learn to meet those five needs in a way that deepens us, and it works with monogamy, then that's great. But I also think that each one of us has our own blueprint, and maybe you're supposed to be monogamous, and maybe somebody else is supposed to not be monogamous, and part of our journey in this life is to find out what's true.

What do you see as the full potential of orgasm?

Orgasm is the most profound human technology that exists. It changes the way we respond to sensation; it changes our brains. It strengthens the parasympathetic nervous system ("rest and digest") as opposed to the sympathetic nervous system ("fight or flight"). Orgasm affects our metabolism, heart rate, blood pressure, respiration, and brain chemistry, and brings about a state of extended deep relaxation. Similar to other mindfulness practices like meditation and yoga, these changes make it possible to develop attention and access flow states—the ability to be "in the zone."

> *Orgasm is the most profound human technology that exists.*

Orgasm also shifts our center of intelligence from the cortex system to the limbic system—which allows us to feel things like intimacy and empathy, and which has a flexible capacity—expanding our appetite for connection. It bolsters "happy hormones"—like oxytocin, dopamine, and prolactin. Friends who are scientists have suggested to me that female orgasm may actually exist solely for the purpose of human connection. There are two scenarios in which a woman's body really pumps out oxytocin (often called the bonding hormone): childbirth and orgasm. In terms of biological evolution, it may just be that we need oxytocin in order to keep us bonded to one another, to keep our culture together.

A huge challenge in our culture right now is recognizing and being able to receive people who think differently from us. But we're inherently empathic beings: I'm built to feel you, you're built to feel me, and we're in a feedback loop together. Orgasm increases my capacity to send out positive frequencies, but also to take you in. It develops empathy, which is such an underrecognized necessity for humans. If I have empathy, I can't hurt you, because I can sense you as part of who I am, as opposed to something separate and removed from me. We have all these big ideas about how to heal the world with this and that program, but we aren't doing the fundamental work of coming to feel one another.

To date, we have been squandering the orgasm impulse. We have been using it, haphazardly, recreationally, to blow off steam, when, if channeled correctly, it could be used to light up the entire power grid of connection. We generally take orgasm outside of this empathic context and serve a toxic mimic of what it really is. Orgasm is so, so much more than the brief, fleeting climax we have been taught to think of it as. When we harness our sexual energy, we change the whole of our lives and become more empathetic, connected, loving human beings. My vision is that we move orgasm into the domain of a practice—where we're cultivating ourselves, our consciousnesses, and our capacity to feel another human being.

If we can make this shift, I think that orgasm will, in a way, take over the world.

CHAPTER 28

experiencing orgasm

Ironically, a lot of advice about how to have THE MOST MIND-BLOWING ORGASM OF YOUR LIFE...can make it harder to do so. Why? Sex therapist and psychology professor Laurie Mintz says there are two things that never mix well: sex and pressure. (And yet, sometimes we just can't help ourselves from asking the question and clicking on the headlines...) Per usual (you can flip back to Mintz's Q&A's on orgasm equality on pages 158–166), she brilliantly satisfies our burning desire to know how to have that mind-blowing orgasm (and maybe a few in a row) without playing into false hype or putting on the pressure.

Taking the Pressure Off

LAURIE MINTZ, PHD

What defines orgasm?

To understand orgasm (male and female), one needs to understand engorgement: Both women and men have erectile tissue in their genitals. For example, women's erectile tissue is located in their inner lips and the inside and outside parts of the clitoris (yes, the clitoris is both an internal and an external organ). There are special capillaries in erectile tissue; when someone is aroused, these capillaries let the blood in but not out, which creates tension that builds up to a very high point. An orgasm is when powerful, rhythmic muscle contractions release that tension. The muscles that contract in women are the pelvic floor muscles—three layers of fourteen muscles that surround a woman's urethra, anus, and vaginal opening. These muscle contractions prevent additional blood from coming into the erectile tissue. When the contractions cease, blood flows in and out again, rather than just in, and erectile tissue shrinks back to its original size and color.

An orgasm is often accompanied by fast breathing and flushed skin on your chest and stomach—and, stating the obvious, having an orgasm feels good. How exactly women experience this buildup of tension and release varies, as does the experience of orgasm from one encounter to another. Many women feel the intense, pulsing muscle contractions of orgasm, yet others feel a general buildup of muscle tension followed by a very pleasurable feeling of overall release. Some orgasms feel intense and some feel diffuse. An

> *An orgasm can feel like riding a series of waves or like being part of one huge tidal wave. Some people experience orgasms as a loud bang, others as a whisper.*

orgasm can feel like riding a series of waves or like being part of one huge tidal wave. Some people experience orgasms as a loud bang, others as a whisper.

Differences in intensity of orgasms can be attributed to physical factors (such as fatigue, length of time since last orgasm, the amount of buildup to this orgasm) and emotional factors (like overall mood, relation to partner, expectations, and feelings about the experience).

How big is mental preparation/anticipation?

Some women need this more than others, and some women need this more at some times than others, but it can never hurt. I encourage women to fantasize about sex, watch or read erotica, or whatever else they want to do to "get themselves in the mood." It's also important to know that for some women, there isn't a linear progression from "feeling horny" to having sex. Instead, some women engage in sex for reasons other than feeling horny (e.g., it will bring them closer to their partner; they know they will enjoy it once it gets going). In fact, some women need to reverse the "get horny, have sex" equation and, instead, have sex to get horny. For these women, mental preparation, anticipation, and fantasy are especially important.

Is the idea that some intercourse positions trump others just hype?

Our culture has distorted perceptions of what "real sex" is (i.e., intercourse), and puts too much pressure on women. The message we get from magazine headlines like "The Best Sex Position for Her Orgasm" is that women "should" orgasm during intercourse—even though some women can't and require more direct clitoral stimulation (oral sex, vibrator, manual stimulation) apart from intercourse. These women are more likely to find pleasure in a turn-taking model. As one example, a partner could give her oral sex until she has an orgasm, followed by intercourse (or something else).

If tips about positioning work—whether it's "woman on top," "coital alignment technique," or putting a pillow under the small of a woman's back or her rear during missionary-style intercourse—it's generally because the woman involved is getting her clitoris stimulated by rubbing or grinding it against a part of the man's body, typically his penis or pubic bone. It can also help if the intercourse position closely mimics the one you use when pleasuring yourself (e.g., on your back or on your stomach). Overall, research finds that women who receive a variety of stimulation during a sexual encounter (kissing, oral sex, manual stimulation, intercourse) are the most likely to orgasm.

FROM THE GOOPASUTRA
WE TRY NOT TO TAKE IT TOO SERIOUSLY

While pressure is not good for your sex life, sometimes a little bit of humor before, during, or after an intimate moment is. Like the classic head-butt in missionary? Whenever it happens, one GOOP staffer told us, "I don't know why, but I can't stop laughing."

Often, though, it's hard to find the humor during a slipup in bed, and it's with time that those occurrences develop into stories that you look back on and laugh about with your partner—usually they're much funnier to you guys than anyone else, doubling the bond between you (e.g., a story from the GOOP files involving accidentally hurting a partner, which our staffer promises is funny now, but that others wouldn't describe as so—we'll save you the decision).

Another person in the office was the casualty: She was having sex in an unfamiliar bedroom (at the Paris Hotel in Vegas) and things got rowdy: "We had just gotten back together and this was the makeup." Well, she got flipped off the bed and came about an inch from cracking her head on the bed's footboard. Again, as she says, "funnier to both of us in hindsight."

Then there are some stories that you enjoy precisely because the other person is no longer in the picture: "I've only had one one-night stand," a GOOP colleague told us. "I snuck out in the middle of the night—after the other person started farting incessantly in their sleep. I was so desperate to get out that I left my bra and favorite pair of hoop earrings. RIP."

Other stories are more humorous to entirely outside parties: A GOOP staffer—having spent Sunday evening as part of an impromptu threesome—was seen running through Paris to the high-speed Eurostar station (Louis Vuitton bag in hand) to meet GP in London one Monday a.m., looking the worse for wear. A friend who broke the sink in a restroom while occupying it with a partner, thereby flooding the entire restaurant—she says she was sitting on the sink and they were "just making out." Another friend, who, trying to be sexy, while actually incredibly nervous, literally asked a guy, "Do you have a license for that equipment?" (They didn't see each other again.)

On the other hand, what begins as a joke could turn into something steamier: One GOOP staffer said she bought a cheesy pair of NFL lingerie in her boyfriend's team colors—rhinestones, the whole deal—intending to be funny. Surprise, surprise: "It was a big hit." She hasn't bought expensive lingerie since. Proof positive that one person's "weird" is another person's "turn-on."

What about multiple orgasms for women?

A multiple orgasm is when you have more than one orgasm during a sexual act, without losing your sense of arousal. (In other words, it isn't having an orgasm, taking a fifteen-minute break, and then starting up again and having another orgasm.) We can roughly categorize multiple orgasms as fitting two general patterns:

- Those that seem to happen one right after the other, without any "downtime" (boom, boom, boom) or buildup between orgasms. Some sexuality experts claim that these are the only true type of multiple orgasms and that they are quite rare. Other sex experts, however, say that these are simply the "reverberations" from the original orgasm or maybe even the continued contractions of one orgasm being perceived as multiple orgasms.

- Those that happen when a woman is restimulated (by herself or a partner) to orgasm a few seconds to a few minutes after the first orgasm. Some sex experts say we shouldn't really call these multiple orgasms, but instead should call these sequential orgasms (I'll use that term here). Sequential orgasms are much more common.

In terms of intensity and pleasure, sometimes the first orgasm will be most pleasurable and sometimes it will be the second, or third, or fourth. There is no set pattern. In my research, I've heard of women who have between two and six orgasms, with a few reports of as many as a dozen. (There was a documentary about a study of five women who could have "super orgasms," defined as more than one hundred in a row, which is obviously very rare.)

There are a lot of myths surrounding the notion of multiple orgasms, with the biggest one being that having them is an important goal to strive for, or that you're missing out if you don't have them. A single orgasm can provide complete satisfaction—many women feel totally "done" after one orgasm, although some may feel the urge for more. Either way, pressure and sex don't mix well—and that includes pressure to "achieve" multiple orgasms.

If interested, how could you experiment with multiple orgasms?

Just as is the case with experiencing orgasms in general, experiencing sequential orgasms seems to become easier for women with time and experience—or, more specifically, as their comfort with and their knowledge of their own bodies grow. Also, like orgasms in general, women are much more likely to have sequential orgasms during clitoral stimulation than during intercourse, including during oral sex or with their own or a partner's fingers or a vibrator.

A few tips if you want to experiment:

- First, as with orgasms in general, you need to actually stop focusing on the goal of having sequential orgasms and fully immerse in the physical feelings you are experiencing. The best way to learn how to do this during sex is to practice it in your daily life through the simple but powerful technique of mindfulness, and then apply that mindfulness to your sex life.

- Most women's clitorises are hypersensitive after having an orgasm, making continued stimulation uncomfortable, even painful. So back off from touching your clitoris and move the stimulation to someplace else on your vulva, such as your inner lips or your mons for a moment or two, even a minute. Alternatively, you could stop touching or vibrating altogether. Some women find that during these moments it helps to continue to rock their bodies or squeeze their pelvic muscles before beginning stimulation again. What's important is that you continue to tune in to your bodily sensations. The urge to have another orgasm may simply arise. Then, follow your body's cues and stimulate yourself again. Some sex experts describe this as "riding the wave," because if you stay in the moment and focus on your physical sensations (rather than turning on your thinking brain), you might find yourself wanting to catch the next wave of arousal.

- If you are one of those rare women who orgasm from intercourse alone, the same principle applies—after the first orgasm, let yourself revel in the sensations and then follow your body's cues and start moving your hips and stimulating your body in ways that feel good.

- I suggest experimenting by yourself first. If you find sequential orgasms are something your body likes or wants, transfer this to partner sex—you'll want to receive the same type of stimulation that you got alone.

What about men and multiple orgasms?

After men ejaculate there is a period of time, called the refractory period, during which it is impossible to have another ejaculation. Most men cannot get another firm erection during this time, which is shorter for younger men than it is for older men. Some younger men will often want to have "another round" after they ejaculate (for example, waiting fifteen minutes and then having another sexual encounter and ejaculating again). This is not the same thing as multiple or sequential orgasms, because the man's arousal decreases between rounds and the second ejaculation is not during the same sex act as the first.

It's rare, but some men can have multiple orgasms (not ejaculations). While orgasm and ejaculation are often considered the same thing (because they almost always occur at the same time), they are actually two distinct events. For men, orgasm is the same as it is for women: strong, rhythmic muscular contractions in the genital area accompanied by very pleasurable feelings. Ejaculation is the release of cum. Men who experience multiple orgasms separate ejaculation and orgasm. Some men always do this and are surprised to learn that others don't. Other men either happen upon or learn this—often during treatment for premature ejaculation, during which they tune in to the feeling of ejaculatory inevitability ("I'm going to come!") and delay that response.

For men who separate orgasm and ejaculation, the most common pattern of multiple orgasm is one or more "dry" orgasms (the plea-surable muscle contractions without ejaculation), followed by one "ejaculatory orgasm" (the pleasurable muscle contractions with the ejaculation). There are also men who reverse this pattern and some who have several of each type with no pattern at all.

There have been two scientific interview studies of these (rare) men, and here is what we know about them: They are generally over thirty-five. During partner sex, their partners stay in a very excited state, which keeps their excitement high. There seems to be an impor-tant biological component—these men have lower levels of the hor-mone prolactin released after ejaculation, which contributes to the refractory period.

Websites and media articles try to teach men to have multiple orgasms, often using the word "edging." Basically, men are encour-aged to separate orgasm and ejaculation and to strengthen their pel-vic muscles to hold their ejaculation back. While some men say they learn this with success, others talk about significant problems occur-ring (for example, blood in their ejaculation). Some sex therapists thus warn men against trying to learn this. To me, it comes back to the bot-tom line of following your own bodily cues—whether you are male or female—and not putting pressure on yourself to "achieve" an orgasm or multiple orgasms. Follow the pleasure wave, not the pressure wave!

CHAPTER 29

the joy of masturbation

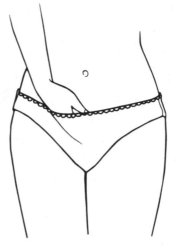

The "fact" that men masturbate is a given in most circles—it's not unusual to have male characters in a TV show, movie, or book talk about masturbating, and the men in our lives do, too. Far less common are conversations among women about masturbating, and references to women masturbating in pop culture—and worse, in sex ed—are still few and far between. And yet we don't know of any sex experts who don't recommend it.

Health and life coach Alexandra Jamieson—author of *Women, Food, and Desire: Honor Your Cravings, Embrace Your Desires, Reclaim Your Body*—refers to masturbation as "self-pleasure" or "sexual self-exploration." She sees it as a practice: "a wonderful, natural way for women to accept themselves on a deep level, and integrate their physical desires while getting to know themselves." She explains the potential benefits, along with how to get started solo (and with a partner) for the uninitiated:

The Ins and Outs of Self-Pleasure

ALEXANDRA JAMIESON

Are there any stats on how often people masturbate?

Masturbation is a natural sexual activity that most people do at some point in their lives. Some people masturbate more than others. There is no "normal" frequency, so if you're worried that you're doing it too often, or not enough—don't. It truly depends on the person.

Broadly speaking, in the National Survey of Sexual Health and Behavior, more than half of women ages eighteen to forty-nine reported masturbating during the previous ninety days. Rates were highest among those twenty-five to twenty-nine, and progressively less in older age groups. About one-third of women in all types of relationships in the sixty- to sixty-nine-year-old cohort reported recent masturbation.

Approximately one-quarter of the men between the ages of eighteen and fifty-nine masturbated a few times per month to weekly. Roughly 20 percent masturbated two to three times each week. Less than 20 percent of men masturbated more than four times a week. Older men were more likely to report no masturbation during the previous year.

For adolescents up to age eighteen and people age seventy and over, masturbation was more common than sex with a partner.

Why do you think masturbation is important for a woman's health?

Masturbation provides so many physical and emotional benefits—we should all consider adding solo self-pleasure time to our calendars as a "well-being" ritual! Women's sexuality has been shamed for so long.

Physical pleasure without food is a wonderful way for women to have a loving connection to their bodies, and masturbation can help us repair our relationship with our physical self.

Many women are concerned about low desire, and masturbation is a great practice for stoking the inner fires. Without pressure to perform for a partner, or worrying about body image, masturbation can increase desire and help you discover what makes you tick, while also bringing you the benefits of orgasm: Orgasm helps the body release oxytocin, the "love and bonding" hormone, which in turn lowers cortisol, the main stress hormone that is chronically elevated in many women (like me!), which can lead to stress eating and weight-loss resistance. Higher levels of oxytocin make us happy and also keep those emotionally triggered food cravings for sugars, cheese, and other "happy foods" at bay.

Hormonally, masturbation is like the best medicine drug companies *wish* they could invent! Oxytocin (O), endorphins (E), and dopamine (D) are released in a woman's body during both pleasurable physical stimulation and at climax, which helps to counter stress hormones. Endorphins ease pain throughout the body, so self-pleasure can help alleviate PMS cramps, as well as other body aches. All three—O, E, and D—help lower stress hormones, which in turn supports cardiovascular health, digestion, and sleep.

> *Hormonally, masturbation is like the best medicine drug companies* wish *they could invent!*

Can you say more about potential emotional benefits?

The emotional benefits of self-pleasure are countless. Many women use "therapeutic masturbation" as a way to increase personal understanding of their own body. This can lead to more and better orgasms, with or without a partner. And more orgasms means more oxytocin, more dopamine, and more endorphins, which all help lower physical and emotional stress.

When women finally take control of their own physical pleasure and experience what climax is like, for and with themselves, they're likely to feel more confident. Women who know what they need to climax because they've practiced by themselves are also going to be able to tell a partner what they like more readily. This can actually help relationships as opposed to degrading them, which is a myth that has been around for far too long.

Are there different benefits for men?

The health benefits of masturbating for men are even more well known, as there's been more funding for studies about men's sexual health. In a 2003 Australian study, men who ejaculated more than five times a week (whether through masturbation or intercourse with a partner) were 33 percent less likely to develop prostate cancer. Men's sperm motility may be improved, as well as the quality and viability of sperm, when they ejaculate more frequently.

Men can also use masturbation in a more conscious way to train themselves to last longer when they do have intercourse with a partner. This is a similar benefit for women: When we know how our bodies work, and what we like, we can better "work" with a partner to get where we want to go!

Are these benefits tied to the end result of orgasm, and/or do you see something else as the goal of masturbation?

Self-pleasure doesn't need to result in climax for it to be helpful, useful, and worthwhile. Simply spending time being very aware and present with your body can help you to increase your self-love. Ultimately, the goal is enjoying *being in* and *experiencing* your body, *for your own pleasure*. Beneficial hormones begin to release, even if climax is not achieved or was not even the goal. Self-soothing through pleasurable touch is a wonderful way to reduce stress, find your center, and even avoid emotionally triggered food cravings. The increase in dopamine and endorphins from self-pleasure hits the same receptors as sugar and other high-impact foods (salt and fat are two big ones). When you enjoy more physical pleasure in your body, you can achieve the same physical pleasure those foods provide.

For women who don't masturbate, how do you suggest getting started?

Perhaps a woman isn't ready to masturbate if she's never tried it, or if she struggles with early messages about shame and sin. Start with making some time to deliberately do what feels good to you, in any way, not just sexually. You might spend quiet, private time taking a bath, enjoying a glass of wine or perhaps some marijuana (if you're in a state where it's legal, of course). You can progress to reading erotica, lounging naked, and caressing your body however feels good to you. Gently exploring some of the sensitive areas of your body with your own hands can be lovely and pleasurable itself. Beneficial hormones are still released with that slight physical pleasure, which can be a beautiful first step.

I also recommend a visit to a sex toy store or website with a knowledgeable female staff (like Babeland). This can help demystify the world of masturbation toys—there's been an explosion in the last few years of toys designed by, and for, women. The most important thing is to take your time, though, and not put pressure on yourself to "do it right." This is for you, so be gentle with yourself and give yourself permission to have pleasure.

What about masturbating with a partner?

For those unfamiliar, mutual masturbation is when you masturbate with or in front of your partner; sometimes you're masturbating at the same time as your partner. Since many of us have been masturbating only in private for our whole lives, it can be nerve-racking to begin.

Just as with solo self-pleasure, mutual masturbation offers the same hormonal benefits, and the oxytocin release can help bond a couple together.

Many of us have been taught that masturbation is "dirty," so doing it in front of someone feels transgressive, which is also what makes it exciting for some of us! Maybe you have some "voyeuristic" fantasies of watching someone else have sex, or perhaps you are more of an "exhibitionist" and want to show off for someone else. Regardless, to get started, first bring it up in a conversation away from the bedroom. Maybe mention you read about mutual masturbation and you'd like to try it, and ask your partner if they'd be into giving it a go.

Ask each other if you have any concerns or boundaries, and then choose a method to get started:

1. One of you can masturbate for the other, showing what you like.
2. You can both masturbate at the same time, lights low, or even off at first. Just knowing you're both engaging together is a nice way to get started.
3. Set a timer, and you can both masturbate for fifteen to twenty minutes with a predetermined end-time. This will take the pressure off and make masturbation the main event as an experiment.
4. One partner can "assist" the other while they handle themselves. Licking, caressing, and other touch can be invited.

What do you make of the normalized conversation around boys/men masturbating, and the lack of one around girls/women masturbating?

Patriarchy. Seriously, it's a social construct that women and girls shouldn't or don't masturbate. Most women and girls do; it's just not as socially accepted or expected that they will. We don't talk about it enough, and I believe we should be teaching girls not just about sexual education, but about *pleasure* education.

In general, sex ed is still focused mostly on pregnancy and sexually transmitted infections. What is missing is the *clitoris*, the only organ in the human body specifically built for pleasure. That is its only function. Most people, including most women, don't even know the whole structure of the clitoris—that it's a large organ, not just a little nub.

What if we taught girls to explore their own bodies and get to know what feels good to them? Might they be better able to ask for what they want, have healthy boundaries, be more likely to engage in sex that was good as opposed to painful or unwanted sex—if they were in touch with what their own bodies were capable of? Might women be more proud and confident in and about their bodies if they knew they were able to bring themselves pleasure?

FROM THE GOOPASUTRA
COMEDIAN LANE MOORE ON OPENING UP THE CONVERSATION

While we're serious about sexual health, sex is clearly better when it's fun—and sometimes it's just plain funny. Lane Moore is an NYC-based stand-up comedian, writer, actor, and musician who has an aptly named interactive comedy show, *Tinder Live*. Moore has a knack for finding humor in varied love and sex subjects, as well as for making these conversations more inclusive and representative of our diverse world. In 2016, Moore won a GLAAD award for her work as a sex and relationships editor with *Cosmopolitan*. Here, she dishes on masturbation and more:

"Social media has definitely allowed women to speak more openly about masturbation than they might IRL, and it's something I tweet jokes about (@hellolanemoore, hi). People are finally realizing that duh, women masturbate, and it's not to turn on dudes; it's for ourselves.

"I always recommend that women just explore their own bodies and see what feels good, because there's not just one way to do it, and you really do have to do a bit of 'research' to figure out what you're into. I knew pretty much immediately that the idea of penetration-only didn't seem to make any sense, and obviously, looking back, I'm, like, *Oh, no shit*. But when you're first getting messages about sex, that's often all you're told, and I think that's why a lot of women get discouraged.

"It always makes me mad that there are so many women in their twenties and thirties, and probably beyond, who don't know how to masturbate in a way that feels great to them. I think so much of changing this is just women allowing themselves to relax and explore in a no-pressure situation. Also, the more varied sources we hear from regarding sex content, the better, because it's not one-size-fits-all, and honestly, it never has been. For one, so many people in my generation and the following generation identify as fluid or queer. It's just a natural progression to open up the dialogue to everyone—it's overdue, really."

PART FIVE

Sex Ed

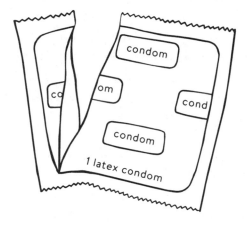

Health class—it's too often still freaking called Health Class, not Sex Class or even Sexuality Class, or Sexual Health Class—generally catalogs every possible unfortunate outcome of a sexual encounter, with none of the upside. Oozing infections and worrying statistics get all the airtime; the details about pleasure and how one might achieve it are left out. So, too, is the female anatomy beyond the uterus and fallopian tubes (for that matter, the sole aspect of male anatomy typically addressed is the penis, and that only in more "evolved" classrooms where students practice squeezing condoms onto bananas). Sexual health of course includes preventing diseases, pregnancy, and exploitation, but a good portion of it is really about optimization. In her book *Girls & Sex*,

Peggy Orenstein compares Holland (where "health class" includes a great deal about pleasure, not to mention relationships) to the United States (where we focus on the negative side effects of sex almost exclusively), and finds that as a result, teenagers and adults report dramatic differences in sexual satisfaction (to make a long story short, the Dutch are satisfied; Americans are not).

Having good sex contributes enormously to our well-being on countless levels, and ensuring that everybody—not, say, one gender, one age group, one race, or any one kind of person—enjoys it can make a difference on a societal level. The personal is political.

So between American health class and porn—the two places where we get most of our information about sex—there's a lot left to learn, from the way that out-of-whack hormones can affect your sex life (and, surprise, the fact that they can be fixed), to nontoxic lube options, how to strengthen your pelvic floor, and the possible link between the prostate and male pleasure. Our expectations around sexual health need to move beyond just potential calamity to its polar opposite—real joy.

CHAPTER 30

clean lube, condoms, and toys

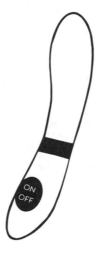

As with any other personal care product, from lipstick to moisturizer to shampoo, the FDA does not regulate the ingredients in lubricant or condoms—and there's no regulation of the materials used to make sex toys. The conventional options for each can contain ingredients/materials that are known toxins. The argument goes that a little bit of a toxin is okay—but this ignores the fact that most people are not using just one product daily; they're using many. (This line of argument also tells us nothing about just how much is safe, or what could happen when these varied toxins interact.) The dose of toxins we're exposed to is much more than what's in a single condom or squirt of lube. The other issue is that some toxins, called endocrine disrupters, might actually be more potent in smaller doses.

When it comes to sex, we're talking about very permeable areas of the body, so we'd much prefer to not split hairs and just be safe, particularly when toxins aren't needed. Condoms are absolutely imperative, lube is often necessary, and sex toys can be wonderful—we just want to choose the cleanest option of each as often as possible. For some guidance, we spoke with naturopathic doctor Maggie Ney, who codirects the Akasha Center for Integrative Medicine in Santa Monica, California.

What's Toxic in the Bedroom?

MAGGIE NEY, ND

What ingredients in lube are a concern?

There are so many choices when it comes to lubricants, and many contain toxic ingredients that are not needed in order for lube to do its job. The vagina and the anus are highly permeable areas, and anything that is applied topically can be absorbed into the body. Read labels as carefully as you read the ingredients in your food.

> *The vagina and the anus are highly permeable areas, and anything that is applied topically can be absorbed into the body. Read labels as carefully as you read the ingredients in your food.*

Parabens, the main toxic ingredient to be aware of, are preservatives, commonly found in most cosmetics (moisturizers, face washes, shaving creams, and lotions). Used to prevent bacterial overgrowth, parabens are known endocrine disrupters, which means they have an estrogenic effect in the body—they bind to the same cell receptors as our own estrogen and interfere with our normal, rhythmic hormonal process. (Parabens have been found inside breast tumor cells. We cannot conclude that parabens cause breast cancer, but we can conclude that our bodies do not efficiently metabolize and eliminate parabens.) Exposure to parabens has been associated with PMS, endometriosis, infertility, low sperm count, and fibroids.

The FDA (which does not regulate what goes into our lubricants) claims that the amount of parabens in our over-the-counter personal care products is too low to pose a toxic effect in the body, and they may be right—if they are referring to a single exposure. The problem is, men and women are applying multiple products to their skin, multiple times a day, every day of the year. With multiple daily use of these products, parabens and other chemicals are accumulating in our bodies, being passed on to our children, and potentially playing a significant role in the health of our reproductive systems.

Other ingredients to be aware of, some of which may be problematic to only some people, include the following:

- Petroleum, like Vaseline, coats the skin, impeding its normal function and changing the pH, which can contribute to vaginal infections.
- Glycerin, a sugar derivative found in many water-based lubricants, can convert to sugar in the vagina. This may contribute to more yeast infections, bacterial vaginosis, and urinary tract infections.
- Propylene glycol is another common ingredient found in water-based lubricants that helps to prevent the lube from drying out. This ingredient is irritating to the skin for some people.
- Chlorhexidine gluconate is a powerful antimicrobial capable of killing healthy vaginal bacteria, which can in turn make women more susceptible to yeast infections, urinary tract infections, and bacterial vaginosis.
- Phenoxyethanol is a tissue irritant for some people.

FROM THE GOOPASUTRA
READING A LUBE LABEL

Avoid personal care products that contain ingredients ending in -paraben (e.g., butylparaben, isobutylparaben, methylparaben, propylparaben). Also, stay away from those with a fragrance: The word "fragrance" can legally conceal hundreds of potentially toxic ingredients a manufacturer doesn't want listed on the label—insist on transparency in labeling. For example, phthalates are potential endocrine disrupters often used in fragrances to make them last longer.

What are the clean lube options?

Personal lubricants can be divided for the most part into three main categories: water-based, silicone-based, and oil-based.

Generally, if it is safe to eat, then it is safe to apply to the skin. Some ingredients that work as a lube are aloe vera, vitamin E, coconut oil, shea butter, olive oil, and almond oil. However, there are certain things to be aware of when it comes to using even the most clean, seemingly safe lubricants.

An organic single-ingredient oil works wonderfully for some people. However, oils degrade latex condoms, compromising their integrity and making them ineffective at protecting against pregnancy and sexually transmitted infections. Also, since these oils are harder to clean off the body (and sheets), they can linger in the vagina and anus, potentially going rancid and causing an odor. (Washing up after use will generally prevent this from happening.) Since the oils are harder to remove, any bacteria that may have been introduced—via your partner's body or a sex toy—have more time to linger and potentially contribute to infections. And coconut oil, for example, has antimicrobial properties, which have the potential to disrupt vaginal flora.

Water-based lube (aloe falls into this category) tends to feel smoother and less sticky than other lubes, and is safe for use with latex condoms and sex toys. Commercially available water-based lubes are more likely to contain parabens and glycerin—so read labels. Lube with a water base is easily absorbed by the skin, so it is simple to clean off but often needs to be reapplied.

Silicone-based lubricants are synthetic and lead to skin irritation in some people. However, this type of lube is often less allergenic than water-based since it has fewer ingredients and is paraben-free. Silicone lube, like water-based lube, is safe for use with latex condoms. It also stays on longer and does not come off in water, which is good for intimacy but not so great for cleaning off our bodies, clothes, and sheets. (Note: Silicone lube also damages silicone toys.)

People will have personal preferences regarding lube consistency and how easy it is to remove from their body and fabrics, and every body is unique and will respond differently to different lubricants. It may take some experimenting to see which safe lubricant works best for you. I see a lot of women in my practice with recurring vaginal infections, and I always want to find the root cause of any chronic issue. Many times I find a lubricant is the trigger of repeated cases of UTIs and vaginal infections, which can be resolved with a simple change.

If you're using a safe lubricant without any side effects, of course continue and enjoy the benefits.

FROM THE GOOPASUTRA
LUBE OF CHOICE

Sliquid is a popular lube brand at GOOP HQ; they make an aloe gel (water-based), with organic extracts (i.e., hibiscus and green tea), that happens to be stain-free and works with latex condoms. Staffers also love Province Apothecary, which makes oil-based personal lubricants (great as long as you aren't using latex with them).

What are the toxicity/allergy concerns when it comes to condoms?

Latex in its purest form is a fluid obtained from the rubber tree. Some people are allergic to latex, which can cause skin irritation, sneezing, runny nose, hives, flushing, and, in very rare situations, anaphylactic reactions. Besides being a potential allergen, natural latex really is not bad for us. The problem is that many companies use chemicals in the processing of the latex. Nitrosamine, for example, is a by-product of latex production. Nitrosamine is a known carcinogen, and while the amount in condoms is very small (less than that obtained from eating a hot dog), it does not need to be in condoms and could be removed without impacting safety and efficacy. Again, because the vaginal walls are so permeable, chemicals are easily absorbed through the walls and into our bloodstream. My concern with people being exposed to even just a small amount of a known harmful chemical is that we are exposed to small amounts of known carcinogens all the time. No one can knowingly say that all of our exposures are safe for everyone. So if there are ways to produce commonly used products safely, without using toxins, we need to start doing it.

Latex is also often treated with casein, a milk derivative. Casein is not toxic, but most people are surprised to learn that their condoms have dairy in them.

Many condoms contain lubricants, too, so we're dealing with the same exposures as outlined for lubes. Some condoms contain the spermicide nonoxynol-9, which is added to kill sperm and sexually transmitted infections. But it is not discriminative in its killing; therefore, with repeated use, it can also disrupt the good vaginal bacteria, which could potentially lead to more bacterial vaginosis and yeast infections. Nonoxynol-9 may also be irritating to the skin of the vagina and the rectum, causing more localized inflammation and a possibly greater susceptibility to contracting sexually transmitted infections like HIV.

Benzocaine and lidocaine are found in many condoms to provide a numbing sensation with the goal of delaying a man's climax, but there are no requirements to label these ingredients on condom packaging. They are not particularly toxic, but people may have a localized reaction and not know they have been added to condoms.

FROM THE GOOOPASUTRA
CONDOMS AND SEXUAL HEALTH

Critical in preventing STDs from HIV to chlamydia, not to mention pregnancy, a big stack of condoms should have a pride of place in just about everybody's nightstand (and makeup bag). Obviously, if you're in a monogamous relationship, your disease- and-pregnancy-prevention options expand dramatically, but many rightly keep them close anyway. Relationships change, you might find a sex toy you love that's better used with a condom (keep reading), and kids become teenagers—like the Girl Scouts (or is it the Boy Scouts?) say: Be prepared. The brand we sell most of on our site is Sustain, which is latex and made free of dyes and fragrances.

What about toys?

There is no regulation of what materials sex toys can be made out of, so companies use whatever ingredients they want—even ingredients that are not allowed in children's toys or pet toys because of their toxic nature. Phthalates, which are probably the biggest issue with sex toys, are added to plastic to keep it flexible and durable. Bendable toys or toys that feel jelly-like probably contain phthalates. Phthalates have been linked to all sorts of health issues including breast cancer, infertility, reduced sperm count, and obesity.

A lot of sex toys are quite absorbent and can harbor mildew, bacteria, and fungus. Generally, the squishier and softer the toy, the more absorbent it is, and the more likely its use could lead to infection. Cleaning these toys well and covering with a condom helps prevent the growth and spread of bacteria and fungus.

The easiest way to pick safe, high-quality sex toys is to purchase them from a trusted manufacturer. Using sex toys made from medical-grade materials is one way to avoid phthalates. These toys are generally made from stainless steel or Pyrex glass. (They have a much firmer feel and tend to be more expensive.)

My overall recommendation is that if you want to experiment with sex toys but don't want to make a big investment, go ahead and experiment and have fun—while being mindful of cleaning them well and keeping them covered when not using. If you end up really enjoying using sex toys and want them to be a part of your life, it is worth learning about and investing in higher quality sex toys made with safe ingredients. They end up lasting longer, so you might save money in the end, and you'll have the peace of mind that comes from using nontoxic and safe materials. Some good, trusted sex toy brands include Fun Factory, Lelo, Fuze, Tantus, Aneros, and VixSkin.

the gender system

W e've arrived at a point in our culture where an understanding that gender is a social construct is expected. But that's simply where the conversation starts: Just because something is created by society doesn't mean it's less real, or without deep significance or complexity—in fact, gender is as important a field of study as it is fascinating. One of the field's luminaries, Susan Stryker—who earned her doctorate in history at Berkeley, completed a postdoctoral fellowship in sexuality studies at Stanford, and is now Associate Professor of Gender and Women Studies at the University of Arizona—knows this well. She's illuminated the often-glossed-over plight of those without cis privilege in her Emmy-winning documentary *Screaming Queens: The Riot at Compton's Cafeteria*, and educated the masses with her introductory textbook *Transgender History: The Roots of Today's Revolution*. Here, she gives us a basic primer on the concept of gender, highlighting nuance where it's mostly unseen, yet almost always present in our daily lives.

Gender Identity and Fluidity

SUSAN STRYKER, PHD

In what way is the concept of gender up for debate?

Gender, like race, is a social system for making meaning out of bodily difference, ranking those differences according to a hierarchy that privileges one kind of body over another, and encouraging us to believe that the hierarchy is in the body, rather than in the social system.

Feminism is the challenging of that hierarchy, based on the knowledge that women don't have to be consigned to the status of "second sex," and that there is nothing "natural" about our subordination.

As the ranking and privileging are entirely social, political change is possible. The gender system changes all the time, in response to different social needs and political demands—what it means to be a woman now bears only a genealogical relationship to what it meant to be a woman for our great-grandmothers. One of the most significant ways gender has changed in recent years is in the increasing willingness to recognize that while humans have two biological sexes, there's no rule that says those sexes have to be the basis for how our society sorts people into the categories we call "men" and "women," no reason that we can't have more than two gender categories, or even that we have to label people based on biology at all.

How is gender cultural?

Gender is highly variable across cultures (and time). The way most readers of this book likely think about gender—that there are two biological sexes called "male" and "female" that are synonymous with two social genders called "men" and "women"—is pretty specific to

European modernity. It's tricky to imagine how we could do things differently. We get tangled up in questions about whether somebody who was born with a capacity to become a sperm-maker can ever "really" be a woman (and vice versa). What needs to be recognized is that being egg- or sperm-makers is not invariably how a society decides who's a man or who's a woman. Most cultures around the world and throughout history have recognized other options.

What does gender have to do with sexuality?

Think of gender identity as a feeling of who you are—a woman, a man, or something else—and sexuality as a sense of who you feel erotic toward. Obviously, gender has something to do with sexuality, because most of us feel erotic toward some genders but not others, which has something to do with our own gender identity. You can't say you are heterosexual, homosexual, bisexual, or pansexual if you haven't already decided who's a man and who's a woman, as well as what you yourself are.

Is there an age when the concept of gender typically takes hold, and we either accept it on some level or feel it's off?

If we think of gender as a social system, one that predates our own individual existence, it's like a soup—or GOOP!—that we come to consciousness inside of, and stay inside of all our lives. There's no experience we have that doesn't take place within a gender context and that isn't shaped by gender. It's kind of like language—there's no thought we have that isn't shaped by language, and how we express our ideas and feelings depends on the languages we know how to speak. If we think about gender as an identity, we can think of it as an acceptance of how we have been positioned in our culture's gender system. Most people don't give this positioning a second thought, and it feels totally natural to consider yourself to be the kind of person your culture tells you that you are.

But some people feel they are not positioned properly, and as a result they experience a lot of distress, sadness, anger, and frustration because of other people not understanding them as they understand themselves. Some people become aware of those feelings of "lack of fit" early on, around age five or even younger—pretty much as soon as they recognize that the world is divided up into different kinds of people, and that they are considered one kind of person rather than another kind. Others might take longer to figure out what's bothering them.

In what ways is gender fluid, and in what ways is it not?

I think it's really idiosyncratic, really personal, what parts of gender feel fluid and what parts feel fixed. First, it's important not to conflate gender (what kind of person are you—man, woman, or other?) with sex (what's your potential biological reproductive capacity—egg, sperm, or neither?). Our cultural belief is that sex is fixed rather than fluid, but even biology is more diverse, and more malleable, than we tend to assume. Some people have a really fluid sense of gender, not identifying too rigidly with being either a woman or a man, while some people have a pretty fixed sense of gender—which might lead you to either stay the gender you've been assigned at birth, or change publicly to the one you consider yourself to be.

But the most important fluidity, in my opinion, is the recognition that it's our culture that decides what our bodies mean. In theory, we can be totally fluid in how we construct gender, and we are constrained only by our imaginations. In practice, creating a new range of gender possibilities requires political activism to tear down all the economic and social arrangements that profit in some way from ranking all bodies and subordinating some of them in ways that enable exploitation, violence, foreclosed life-opportunities, and unequal rates of death.

How can we change the way we talk about gender?

It's vital to recognize the difference between biology and social category, and between sense of self and culturally defined labels for kinds of people. The fact that it takes egg and sperm to make a new little human is not going to change anytime soon, but even far-out, science fiction–sounding scenarios involving advanced reproductive technologies and artificial genomes are not completely beyond imagining. Already things like gestational surrogacy (renting one woman's womb to grow a baby from two other persons' genetic material) are transforming how we manage childbirth and make families. But quite apart from how we increasingly intervene technologically in the biology of reproduction, we need to acknowledge far more than we do that biology is not in fact destiny when it comes to how we categorize people; how we give different categories of people different legal rights and have different expectations of them, or ask them to shoulder different social responsibilities. We need to cut people way more slack about figuring out how to live in a gendered world.

> *We need to cut people way more slack about figuring out how to live in a gendered world.*

the hormone reset

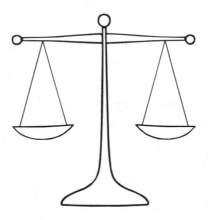

If you're feeling like your body or your sex drive is off-kilter, it's worth checking in with your doctor to see if you have a hormonal imbalance. Author of *Younger, The Hormone Reset Diet,* and *The Hormone Cure*, Dr. Sara Gottfried reports that 70 percent of the low sex drive cases in her practice are hormonal. Other related symptoms of this hormonal imbalance that she commonly sees include lackluster orgasms, sexual boredom, and vaginal dryness. Below she shares an immensely helpful primer on the hormones that influence our libido and sexual health, as well as her tips for keeping them in balance and finding satisfaction in our sex life at every age.

Hormone Balancing and Its Impact on Sex

SARA GOTTFRIED, MD

How do you contextualize the relationship between hormones and our sexual well-being?

When your hormones are in balance— neither too high nor too low—you look and feel your best. You feel lusty, desiring, and desirable, and aligned with your most authentic self. When your hormones are out-of-whack, you may experience a range of symptoms, including fatigue, numbness,

> *Sex is not essential to life, but feeling sexual hunger and wanting sex is a portal to something bigger. How you do sex is how you do everything.*

sugar cravings, weight-loss resistance, trouble sleeping, anxiety or irritability, and stress. Sex is not essential to life, but feeling sexual hunger and wanting sex is a portal to something bigger. How you do sex is how you do everything.

When your sex life is in balance, you automatically find freedom in other areas of life where you may have previously struggled.

I wish low sex drive, which 80 percent of my patients experience, were a quick fix. But the truth is that if you figure out the root cause of why you don't want to have sex, you're going to address something far bigger than sex. It's the basis of healing from the inside out. It's not a matter of new lingerie or a tricked-out topical cream; it's not a bandage for symptoms, but rather a comprehensive functional protocol of medicine that addresses something deeper you may not be able to see or even know exists. With sex in particular, strongly held, unconscious beliefs are often present. In my practice, when low sex drive is addressed on this level, there are other downstream benefits of healing one's relationship with sex. You feel whole. You don't crave wine... It takes work, you have to really want it, and you need to be willing to accept help, but the upshot is that the benefits are sustained.

What are the main hormones that influence our sexual health and libido?

Estrogen, progesterone, oxytocin, cortisol, thyroid, and testosterone are the hormones that impact sexual health, all in different ways:

- **Estrogen** makes you feel feminine, present in your body, and caring about your appearance—you can witness estrogen's effects particularly at puberty when it rises and girls obsess about their looks, and again in your forties when dry shampoo and yoga pants seem to be the best options. Estrogen gives you breasts, hips, and a lubricated vulva and vagina.

- **Progesterone** is the counterpart to estrogen; in fact, you want a minimum ratio of 100 progesterone molecules to 1 estrogen molecule for optimal libido (P:E of 100; normal is 100–500), as measured in saliva on day 21 or 22 of the menstrual cycle. Progesterone is soothing, making you less likely to feel anxious about your "imperfect" body parts, or to worry about something irrelevant when it's time for sex.

- **Oxytocin** makes you feel loving, connected, and grounded, like a cashmere hoodie. Due to genetics, lack of sex, or age, you may be running low.

- **Cortisol**, the main sex hormone, can rob you of all of the other hormones. Cortisol is the highest value hormone because it is involved in maintaining your blood pressure, blood sugar, and immune function. If your cortisol is dysregulated, you are likely to make cortisol at the cost of other sex hormones, especially progesterone and testosterone.

- **Thyroid.** Think of your thyroid as an environment-sensing organ. If your body's burden of toxins is too high, or you keep driving an autoimmune attack of your thyroid by eating a lot of gluten, you may have little interest in sex.

- **Testosterone**, finally, may be the most direct hormone involved in sex drive for men and women. Women have 10 times less testosterone than men, but that means we're exquisitely sensitive to changes. I think of testosterone as the hormone of vitality, confidence, and agency, all of which we need to remain sexually awake and engaged.

How do imbalances in these hormones manifest?

There are many manifestations of hormonal imbalance. For some of my patients, hormone imbalance shows up as weight gain; for others, as gut issues or a lack of stress resilience; but for 80 percent, it presents as low sex drive, lackluster orgasms, sexual boredom, or vaginal dryness.

Many women don't know that hormonal imbalances cause them to feel depleted and unsexy. In my years of clinical practice, I've seen it all: Women who feel their bodies have turned against them. Women who would rather mop the floor than have sex with their partners. Women who wonder if they are just a low-libido type and try to get sex over with as quickly as possible. Women who wonder if they can still have a happy marriage if they are honest about never wanting sex again.

Before you think you have a moral failing when it comes to sex and desire, please ask your doctor to check your hormone levels. They are the cause of 70 percent of the cases of low sex drive in my practice. I think of low libido as reflecting a complex inner state, one that usually lacks the homeostasis the body craves. In all cases of low libido, I find that the cortisol level is off, and since it's the boss of your other hormones and a top priority (you need it to survive because it governs blood sugar and blood pressure), you have to fix it first. Hormones can generally be fixed with proper lifestyle adaptations—particularly dietary changes, smart exercise, detoxification, and natural hormone balancing.

Is there any sex drive without hormones?

While hormones are an important part of a healthy sex life, they aren't everything. In functional medicine, we think not just of the health condition (e.g., low sex drive) but also the *terroir* or context of the health condition—the soil; that is, the relationship and whether it needs to be cleared; the history of sex; the level of stress and status of the control system for hormones (the hypothalamic-pituitary-adrenal-thyroid-gonadal axis); the structure and function of the involved organs; the communication system; the detoxification process; as well as other emotional, spiritual, and mental components.

I'd say there is sex drive without hormones in outliers: I have some patients who are very happy with their sex lives after menopause even though their hormones are close to zero, but they had a strong libido and sexual connection before their hormones waned. To me, these women exemplify the adage "Use it or lose it." If you're regularly using your sexual organs (eyes, mouth, breasts, skin, vulva, clitoris, vagina), you're less likely to have low sex drive. More commonly, I help women regain their missing sex drive after a hormonal hit, such as having a baby, surgical or natural menopause, breast cancer, or aromatase inhibitors.

What kind of hormonal testing do you recommend?

I have a free questionnaire online (thehormonecurebook.com/quiz/) that will help you get an initial assessment of common symptoms and the hormone imbalances that are likely to underlie them. Record your symptoms and check in with your physician.

Below are the tests I most commonly recommend for my functional medicine patients:

Basic:

Request the following blood tests (fasting 12 hours before) from your doctor:

- Cortisol

- TSH, free T3, reverse T3, free T4 (to check thyroid)
- DHEA
- Testosterone: free, bioavailable, and total
- Glucose and hemoglobin A1C (a 3-month summary of your blood sugar)
- If overweight, fasting insulin
- ALT (to check liver)
- If still cycling:
  - Day 3 estradiol
  - Day 3 FSH
  - Days 21–23 progesterone
- If menopausal:
  - Estradiol
  - FSH

Advanced:

Consider the Complete Hormones profile test from Genova Diagnostics or the DUTCH test from Precision Analytical. These tests will tell you more about your adrenals (both short- and long-term function), and your estrogen metabolism, which will help you determine if you have too much wear and tear from cortisol. They will reveal your anabolic-to-catabolic ratio—whether you have enough growth-and-repair hormones (e.g., testosterone) to balance out the wear-and-tear hormones (e.g., cortisol). These two tests also shed light on things like whether you have a modifiable tendency toward breast cancer or not, or a risk of osteoporosis. Review the results with your doctor (ideally an informed, collaborative, functional medicine clinician).

What's the effect of birth control hormones?

Birth control pills (BCPs) contain synthetic versions of estrogen and progesterone, the two main female hormones. When taken as an oral contraceptive, these hormones prevent ovulation, thicken the lining of the cervix to prevent sperm from reaching any eggs that might have been released, and thin the uterine lining to make it harder for a fertilized egg to implant. The pill "tricks" the female body into not having a normal monthly cycle, which prevents unwanted pregnancy in the range of 99.6 percent for error-free users and 91 percent in typical users. In scientific terms, BCPs inhibit ovulation by suppressing your production of luteinizing hormone (LH). BCPs decrease your testosterone levels, and may cause low sex drive, vaginal dryness, and painful intercourse.

Over time, the dose of synthetic estrogen in BCPs has declined, more synthetic progestins have been included, and regimens beyond the 21-day active/7-day placebo have been developed and marketed. Along with these changes, BCPs have gone far beyond pregnancy prevention. As you probably know, BCPs are prescribed, mostly off-label, for acne, hirsutism, painful periods (dysmenorrhea, including endometriosis), irregular menstruation, heavy periods (menorrhagia), reduction in risk of ovarian and endometrial cancers, and improvement in premenstrual syndrome (PMS) and premenstrual dysphoric disorder (PMDD).

BCPs reduce acne and hirsutism by lowering your testosterone levels, but sometimes your testosterone can drop too much, potentially leading to new symptoms. Studies show that free (or biologically available) testosterone levels drop on average by 61 percent in women on BCPs. It's thought that BCPs increase by fourfold the level of sex hormone binding globulin (SHBG), which acts like a sponge that soaks up testosterone. Approximately 25 percent of women on BCPs have decreased lubrication, vaginal dryness, and lack of arousal. Furthermore, 5 percent of women experience painful sexual relations. Two things trouble me about these results: First, many women don't realize the problems are a side effect of BCPs, so they don't seek help. Second, when you stop the BCPs, you don't necessarily go back to normal. In fact, up to one year later, your testosterone levels may still be out of balance. Finally, birth control pills are associated in multiple studies with an increased risk of breast cancer, including a 2017 study from the *New England Journal of Medicine*.[1]

I was never taught to counsel patients about these risks, but now I believe they should be part of full informed consent. BCPs are not the agent of feminism I once thought they were—lowering your testosterone can reduce confidence and agency. I grit my teeth as I say it, but I consider oral contraceptives the biggest hormonal problem for women, caused by doctors who do not provide full informed consent. Yes, women benefit from avoiding the alternative of an unwanted pregnancy or even ovarian cancer, but over my years of practice, I've seen many women suffering from the side effects of these pills—including vaginal dryness, lost libido, micronutrient deficiency, early menopause, and worsening mood.

What's the first step toward resetting your hormones?

It is absolutely possible for you to reset your hormones, and lifestyle changes play a huge role in how your body handles hormonal changes. I take a food-first philosophy—you want a foundation of nutrient-dense whole foods. To fuel your body to work at optimal levels, I suggest you eat mostly plant-based foods and more foods that detoxify your body—such as cruciferous vegetables, fruits, and nuts. Plus, eating more vegetables helps to lower estrogen and cleanse out the gut: The fiber lowers blood sugar and insulin, and has a direct effect on the good bacteria in the gut, which allows you to follow the golden rule of estrogen—use it, then dump it.

The connection between meat and estrogen is profound, so go easy on animal-based foods—think of meat as a complement to your plant-based dishes. When you eat conventionally raised red meat, estrogen overload is more likely. When you go meatless, your estrogen decreases. Not surprisingly, vegetarians have the edge here. This could be due to the hormones in the meat, the type of bacteria cultivated in the guts of people who eat a lot of meat, or a combination of factors. We do know that a meat-based diet is linked to higher body mass index and that too much of the wrong type of saturated fat raises estrogen. When you reverse your estrogen dominance, you clear the path toward a healthy weight and reduce the incidence of estrogen-dominant conditions such as diabetes, metabolic syndrome, and certain forms of breast, ovarian, and endometrial cancers.

If you're estrogen is out-of-whack, limit yourself to 18 ounces or less per week of grass-fed red meat in order to prevent estrogen overload. (Grass-fed beef has higher levels of omega-3s than grain-fed beef, which is problematic for those who are estrogen-dominant.) Definitely skip the processed meat like sausage, hot dogs, deli meats, and bacon, as well as meat from concentrated animal feeding operations (CAFOs).

Avoid processed foods, especially unrefined carbohydrates that can worsen adrenal problems, and cut out sugar and sugar substitutes. Eating refined carbohydrates contributes to high insulin (insulin resistance) and low testosterone, thereby depositing more fat. Limit carbohydrates to only the slow carbohydrates that won't spike your insulin, such as those in sweet potatoes, yams, pumpkin, and quinoa. Minimize grains and dairy, or skip them altogether if you need to lose weight or if you want to lower cortisol.

Curb unnecessary inflammation by avoiding foods most likely to cause intolerance; gluten and dairy are the biggest culprits. Reduce alcohol and caffeine consumption to reset cortisol levels, relieve mood swings, and vamp up your energy levels.

Beyond diet, what's important?

Sleep, stress, supplement. Restorative sleep will put you on a track to better health and more balanced hormones. When you make sleep a priority, you put your growth hormone production back in high gear and power your hormones to work for you.

Try coping differently with stress. Develop a more playful attitude: laugh more, roll with the punches, hang out with girlfriends, or take a superhot detox bath with Epsom salts. Find ten minutes to meditate, or practice yin yoga—over time meditation resets cortisol levels, raises serotonin, lowers inflammation, and improves cognitive function including attention. These activities will serve as a buffer for you,

THE HORMONE RESET | 219

especially if you're a highly sensitive person, and may help keep cortisol in the green zone. You'll feel a noticeable difference right away once you start implementing better strategies to care for yourself, and relax.

Last, you can use supplements to fill in any gaps and address specific issues. For example, to aid with lower estrogen levels, I recommend the herb maca. Maca has been shown to increase estradiol levels in menopausal women, and helps with depression, memory, concentration, energy, and vaginal dryness. Vitamin C and chasteberry help to normalize progesterone in the body. Phosphatidyl serine improves cortisol levels and lean body mass.

How do we balance the potential health risks of taking hormones vs. the need to reset for sexual well-being?

I ask all of my patients: Are you satisfied with your sex life? Do you have sex with men, women, or both? Then, most importantly, how do you prioritize your sexual well-being right now in your life? Is something missing? Do the potential health risks of taking hormones bother you? It's really about quality of life, and I want you to feel empowered to make an informed decision that is most suitable for your life.

There are many ways to recruit natural methods to balance your hormones before resorting to prescription bioidentical hormone therapy. I have a three-step protocol for each hormone: Step 1—start with targeted lifestyle changes and supplements for four to six weeks, and if you're not feeling better, move on to step 2, herbal therapies. For instance, maca is shown to improve libido in women in perimenopause and menopause. Make yourself a daily maca shake, and if you don't feel better after four to six weeks, then move on to step 3, bioidentical hormones.

The bioidentical hormones that tend to trip up most women long-term are estrogen, progesterone, and especially testosterone. So we discuss the risks, benefits, and alternatives to taking them before I prescribe. Topical estrogen cream, such as estriol or estradiol, is usually the easiest to accept since the data are rigorous and show long-term safety.

When it comes to testosterone, I wish we had robust outcome data on exactly what it means to your health long-term to restore testosterone to a physiological level, but the longest trials we have are six months.

My patients sometimes choose to take a hormone as an experiment—they try it for six weeks and see what happens to their libido. We recheck their blood levels at six weeks, and adjust accordingly so that they're in the optimal range (the top half of the normal range for free or bioavailable testosterone). My patients respond in one of three ways: They love it, start swinging from the chandeliers, and decide they accept the risks because their quality of life is better. Or they are in the optimal physiological range and realize they don't like their partner. Or they find taking hormones too high-maintenance and worrisome, and prefer a quieter sexuality. Most of my patients who take hormones fall into the first camp.

Can you talk about the emotional element of hormonal changes?

Emotional upheaval is a telltale sign of hormonal imbalance. For instance, when estrogen levels are high in relation to progesterone, women often experience a wild ride of emotions before their periods.

Your hormonal system communicates with your mind and the rest of your body as a complex and sophisticated neuroendocrine communication network, or dashboard, that encompasses your brain chemicals and hormones. Specific parts of your brain—essentially, your hypothalamus and pituitary, which are part of your limbic system—control this network.

Here's the problem: One part of your brain tends to exert more influence than any other, and that's your amygdala, where you take in stress, interpret, and then embed news and stimuli from your environment, and manufacture your mental and emotional state. Women ages thirty-five to fifty have a tendency to overrespond emotionally to triggers in an immediate, reactionary, and sometimes overwhelming manner. There's a mismatch between the trigger and the response. I know, because I've been there, and I see many women each day in my office who feel this way. Here's how one woman describes it:

> I'm so up and down with my emotions. They're right at the surface. Discernment? Gone. Some days at work, I'm on my game and can keep it together, and other days, I burst into tears for no good reason. It's not cool when that happens at work. It's also not just before my period, although my reactions are certainly amplified at that time. I just can't trust myself anymore to have my act together.

It is very difficult to manage the amygdala, yet it impacts your levels of critical hormones, such as cortisol, estrogen, progesterone, and thyroid. The amygdala, hypothalamus, and pituitary organize, integrate, and coordinate what you're interested in, mood, fertility, sexual desire, skin texture, general aging, and weight via neuroendocrine communication. Your brain determines hormone levels throughout the body, and, reciprocally, hormone levels direct brain activity through feedback loops—and the dance between the two determines your ability to feel optimal vim and vigor.

What kind of hormonal changes are natural as we age vs. those that indicate something else is up?

Nothing annoys me more than a doctor who brushes aside pain points like low libido as simply a "symptom of aging." I believe it is both possible and *important* for a woman to maintain a strong sex drive long past her childbearing years.

To achieve this, a little work is required—keeping balanced hormones, trying some proven botanicals, practicing a little self-love, and employing a steady diet

I believe it is both possible and important *for a woman to maintain a strong sex drive long past her childbearing years.*

of quality orgasms—but it's more than worth it in the long run. Of course, libido will naturally wax and wane. Ultimately, it's your choice.

It's not normal to hate sex or have no libido, no matter your age. The first step is balancing your hormones if you're feeling asexual. You can also change your sexual routine. You may need to be creative in order to bring in some variety while you're resetting your hormones. My favorite is doing Orgasmic Meditation (OM), a cross between mindfulness and genital stroking, for thirteen minutes [see page 171 for more]. I find that OM is a wonderful practice for people who are tired of sex, or tired of how fat they feel, or just plain *tired*. It fills your tank with oxytocin, and we all need more of that! In men, oxytocin raises testosterone and lowers cortisol; and in women, it raises estrogen and makes the thyroid work better.

FROM THE GOOPASUTRA
YES, YOUR VAGINA LOOKS FANTASTIC

As much as we love the fact that new, hormone-free technology like vaginal laser treatments has the potential to make sexual wellness easier for millions of women, we don't love the simultaneous push toward more "aesthetic" vaginas through some of the same technologies. Now, when you're done obsessing over your thighs and your breast size and the shape of your face, you can turn your insecurities further inward, toward your very core—and reshape an area designed for your pleasure.

There are a number of factors at work here: People often blame porn, the aesthetics of which can be mind-numbingly uniform, between the extreme close-ups and anal bleaching... But gynecologists began getting more "Is my vagina normal?" complaints as bikini-line grooming and especially the "full Brazilian" look took hold across the nation: There's just a whole lot more to look at when you've got no pubic hair. All of a sudden, the average person is seeing more of the exterior of the vagina (theirs and other people's) than ever before in history—in porn and in life. Then add in the new availability of surgical "fixes" for the way our vaginas look, and you have a new vehicle for female self-loathing. Depending on what "procedure" a person has done (never mind how much they pay for it), it can also be a form of serious self-mutilation, but even less-draconian measures— not kidding, there's now a tastefully packaged line of vagina "makeup" on the market—send a crazy-making message: that our vaginas are there to be seen, not to feel, not to function.

The Labia Library is one brilliant solution: It's pictures of many, many women's vaginas. As with penises, the variety is huge—and somehow, all versions have managed to attract repro-ductive partners over millennia. Spend some time on that site, and you'll internalize the truth: that "normal" doesn't have strict parameters. Beyond that, consider pubic hair (it's back, even in porn), consider the beauty inherent in the pleasure your vagina brings you, and…use it more. Masturbate, have sex—enjoy.

Notes

1. Mørch, LS, et al. "Contemporary Hormonal Contraception and the Risk of Breast Cancer." *New England Journal of Medicine* 2017; 377:2228–2239. http://www.nejm.org/doi/full/10.1056/NEJMoa1700732.

sex and aging

As we learn more about the ways sexual well-being directly affects our health, we start to understand how critical it is to look for the unaddressed, unspoken challenges: Aging changes human sexual function in both sexes, and not speaking of it or denying it leaves millions feeling frustrated and alone. The patient-doctor relationship is proven, in practically every area of health, to have a profound effect on treatment outcomes, so finding practitioners to help us navigate both the physical and the mental aspects of our sometimes dramatically (and sometimes not) changing bodies is important. Physician's assistant Virginia Reath, who has a master's in public health and sex education, has practiced reproductive and sexual health for more than thirty-five years. She helps women of all ages navigate sexual health and well-being through the lenses of naturopathic medicine, nutrition, herbalism, and bioidentical hormone therapy, as well as conventional medicine, in her NYC offices. She works in conjunction with gynecologists to address her patients' issues, questions, and overall health; here, she talks about perhaps the most significant issues for many of them: sex and getting older.

How Sexuality Changes Through Perimenopause, Menopause, and Beyond

VIRGINIA REATH, RPA, MPH

What's the most important message women need to hear about sex and aging?

However dire hormonal changes may sound, they do not have to be reasons to avoid or reject being sexual. Sexuality is a force within us that we are born with and we die with. It is "the smile within."

Numerous treatments are available for the physical changes aging brings to our sexuality, but it's important to recognize that there are many factors other than hormones that affect women, sex, and aging. It is not only physical changes, but also cultural and psychological pressures that influence how women experience aging. We need a consciousness that promotes positive radical aging and respects all people; and we need a movement to resist body self-hatred and shame. Women specifically also need more support and permission to pay attention to nourishing their own sexual and emotional needs.

How can aging—particularly perimenopause and menopause— affect our sex lives and sexual health?

For some women, menopause and perimenopause mimic a second puberty, with all the expectations, anticipations, and fears rolled into one. The initial upset of hormonal balance prior to the actual onset of menopause is often the most confusing and bewildering time. After years of living in, and being accustomed to, one's body, even a gradual shift in how that body works can be disconcerting.

During perimenopause, a woman's menstrual cycle or flow, her moods, and her energy may all subtly change. Periods become irregular; emotions become unpredictable. For some women, this time is marked by increased anxiety, disrupted sleep, hot flashes, and changes in libido. For others, perimenopause feels like prolonged PMS.

When the established relationship with one's own body is altered, it creates a sense of dissonance or internal upheaval. This change may be so stressful, so intimately tied up in one's own sense of self, that it becomes a source of shame or guilt. This can be compounded if the healthcare people seek out only medicalizes their lives and if there is a lack of assistance in coping physically and emotionally. When women feel dismissed and are having a challenging time finding the help they need from medical providers, this often worsens the sense of emotional, mental, or physical burden.

As we age, fat is redistributed around the mid belly and thighs, and we tend to gain five to ten pounds per decade. Since we live in a fat- and weight-phobic society, this sets women up to feel more fear and shame, which can of course affect their sex lives—some may even avoid sex altogether, regardless of their hormone health. This sexual body shame interrupts and steals so much pleasure and love between people. We can be our worst critics, leading to a tendency to isolate ourselves from the joy of connection with another physically, and the fear of being sexual. Some patients report to me that they even stop masturbating because they don't want to desire something they fear they cannot have.

What are symptoms of actual menopause, and how do they affect us?

There are such varied reactions to menopause from woman to woman. For some, it can feel like only a flush here and there, while for others it feels like a frightening cascade of dramatic symptoms: sweats, unpredictable flashes of heat, flushing of the face, insomnia, depression. Many women do not suffer at all through menopause, but for those who do, there is help—and no shame in seeking it. (Note: An important health condition that too often goes misdiagnosed in women over forty is thyroid disorders. The symptoms can mimic menopausal changes, so it is very important to have a thyroid screening.)

Life itself is often more challenging during the time menopause is occurring: From marriage, divorce, relationships with adolescent children, aging-parent responsibilities, and financial concerns, to the potential aches and pains of physical aging—the disruption caused by menopause can challenge even the strongest of women. Add to this mix the changes in the sexual response cycle and vaginal tissue, and you can imagine why our stress hormones begin escalating exponentially as our sex hormones decrease.

The effects of the hormonal battle alone can be exhausting: Daily life often becomes harder to manage as symptoms—including mood swings, hot flashes, night sweats, trouble sleeping—become more pronounced. The effects can leave one feeling physically depleted, potentially resulting in adrenal fatigue and a sense of being overwhelmed. Menopause is a time in a woman's life to feel her power, wisdom, and sexuality, but the persistent haze of shame that surrounds this physiological transition turns our focus away from the strengths of women and their sexual intelligence.

Menopause is a time in a woman's life to feel her power, wisdom, and sexuality, but the persistent haze of shame that surrounds this physiological transition turns our focus away from the strengths of women and their sexual intelligence.

Why does sex often change as we age?

The vagina is the most estrogen-rich area of the human female body, so it is here that the lack of hormones—estrogen, specifically—is often most apparent after the onset of menopause: The vulva becomes thinner, losing its fat pad on the mons and labia. Vaginal mucosal membranes become less lubricated and less able to stretch. The labial and clitoral hood becomes thinner and dry. The entrance or vaginal cuff where the labial skin becomes the internal vaginal tissue can become painful during penetration. The vaginal ridges that women have to decrease the friction of penetration flatten and become smooth in menopause, which can make intercourse and penetration uncomfortable or painful.

All these changes affect not only penetration with sex, but masturbation as well. Clitoral stimulation may become more irritating than pleasurable, due to the sensitivity of the dryer, thinner skin that surrounds the clitoris. Orgasm, as well as the intensity, frequency, and ease of arousal all begin to feel very different. If women are having fewer orgasms, the blood flow to the vulva and vagina decreases, which can compound the issue of dryness. (Though testosterone also decreases at the onset of menopause, it's effect on libido and orgasm as woman age is still unclear, and seems to vary from woman to woman.)

What are the best solutions for symptoms of depleted vaginal estrogen?

Several treatments help remoisturize, lubricate, and restore estrogen to the tissues, though until very recently the only medical treatment was the use of vaginal estrogen and lubricants. There are herbal remedies that can help as well: vitamin E oil, coconut oil, olive oil, shea butter, aloe vera, Aloe Cadabra, oil of primrose, hyaluronic gel, progesterone and DHEA vaginal cream/suppositories, black cohosh, and calendula. (It is important to remember that condoms can break or tear when used with oils.)

Lubricants help with the glide factor of penetration [see page 199 for a GOOP guide to nontoxic lube]. I find silicone lubricants a better option as they create a glide buffer, whereas some water-based lubricants can get sticky and pull on vaginal tissue. Vaginal estrogen is available by prescription as creams, suppositories, and vaginal rings. Often women on systemic hormone replacement therapy (HRT) will benefit vaginally from them, but many women need localized treatment as well; vaginal estrogens do require constant use and application (which some find annoying), along with gynecological follow-up, as they sometimes build up an irregular lining of the uterus.

Vaginal lasers have become a treatment for vaginal dryness and menopausal vaginal pain. The treatment, which usually involves three sessions, stimulates the collagen and increases blood flow to the vaginal tissue inside and out. Vaginal lasers are expensive but appear to really work. They are an optimistic option for many women—especially those who cannot use estrogens at all.

What are the best ways to treat the symptoms of menopause and perimenopause?

Herbs

For centuries, herbs have been used to help manage hormonal changes and transitions, and herbs and supplements are especially useful for women who need support but do not want to take hormones. Many herbs act like a hormone, either progestogenic, estrogenic, or adaptogenic, without being true active hormones—thereby producing positive effects without the high risk. Many excellent supplements and vitamins can be tailored to support optimal health for individual issues. (As mentioned above, thyroid disorders sometimes present as hormonal disorders, so it's important to be checked for them.) I most often prescribe Chaste Tree Berry/Vitex, black cohosh, red clover, extract of rhubarb, B complex, and OTC progesterone cream. For adrenal support and to manage cortisol levels, I may prescribe prod-ucts with maca, Siberian ginseng, ashwagandha, rhodiola, or a combi-nation. Remember: It is very important to get the advice of a provider or practitioner with knowledge of herbs and supplements to be sure you are getting correct dosages and purchasing from a reliable source to ensure authenticity and quality.

Hormone replacement therapy/bioidentical hormones

Conventional medicine has long established that replacing the estro-gen and progesterone that decline in menopause relieves symptoms such as hot flashes, night sweats, insomnia, mood disturbances, vaginal dryness, and painful sex. The aim of HRT (hormone replacement ther-apy) or BHRT (bioidentical hormones) is to restore female hormones to levels that allow the body to function as it did prior to the shifts. Most clinicians choose from prescribed pharmaceutical hormones that are synthesized to mimic or replace the hormones in a woman's body. The prescribed treatments include birth control pills, a hormone-releasing IUD (such as Mirena or Skyla), estrogen, progesterone, and testosterone.

Bioidentical hormone therapy involves restoring and maintain-ing hormonal balance with hormones that are biologically identical to those produced by the body. Bioidentical hormones are synthesized from yams and soy extracts and may include all three types of estrogen (estriol, estradiol, estrone), progesterone, and testosterone, as well as precursor hormones like DHEA and pregnenolone. These are the most commonly prescribed hormones for treatment of menopause.

To match a patient's individual needs, bioidentical hormones are usually custom-compounded by a pharmacy clinician. Since many women in the first stages of hormonal transition need more varia-tion and tweaking in dosing, compounded products make this eas-ier. They are available in different delivery modes including creams, gels, suppositories, oral capsules, and sublingual lozenges, allowing for even more variation in dosing and strength—as opposed to the "one-size-fits-all" approach of conventional prescribed pharmaceutical treatments. As always, talk to your doctor about what is right for you.

We now have better studies and reports of the efficacy and safety of hormone replacement, and current thinking is encouraging on the benefits of HRT and BHRT versus the risks, depending on dose and duration.

How much difference can a toned pelvic floor make as we age?

Pelvic floor awareness and therapy have made a significant difference for those suffering from pelvic pain, urinary, and/or bladder issues due to childbirth, trauma, surgery, and/or sex. Pilates, Kegel exercises, vaginal weights, and certain yoga poses promise a better sex life by strengthening the pelvic floor. Though the benefits of a flexible and strong pelvic floor are well documented, the promise can go overboard. In fact, clinicians are seeing many women with overcontracted pelvic floors (often due to overzealous core exercises and incorrect Kegels), resulting in difficult births and worsening sexual pain. Being able to release the pelvic floor slowly is more important than contracting tighter and tighter. I like to say that the vagina should be more like an oyster, not an oyster cracker!

What's the mistake people make with Kegels? How do you do them right?

I find that many people mistake the butt, groin, and lower stomach muscles for the pelvic floor, and they think that clenching, or even a squeeze and release—e.g., it stops the flow of urine—is a Kegel. But the actual pelvic floor and core muscles are far deeper than that: Think of the pelvic floor as a hammock that needs to be pulled up—not squeezed in and out. If your butt muscles are moving and lifting up and down, that's wrong. The vagina is a canal: You want to pull up from the vaginal entrance toward the sternum, as if you were sucking yourself in to pull up tight pants.

What are some of the consequences of fear of aging you see in your practice?

Cultural norms that perpetuate youth cultivate a dread of aging, and that dread can produce stress that has physiological results. What lies behind so much of the fear of growing old may be shame and embarrassment—and this affects our confidence, our self-esteem, and our physical and mental health. We are deeply influenced by our own body dysmorphias, what we think others see, and the anti-aging bias of our cultural imagery. Being unable to accept our aging—if we are not okay if our thighs sag, or wrinkles deepen, or knees stiffen—may send many of us into hiding from intimacy. Even the best of marriages and relationships are threatened by the sexist historical narrative that partners will inevitably leave, seeking out younger lovers, or more Viagra, or both.

Too many women, when asked if they are sexually active, answer according to whether they have a partner or not. We do not need to be in a couple to find sexual release or pleasure. Not having a partner does not determine whether you are sexually alive. Keeping that "smile within" intact is crucial to being open to connection, which can include physical intimacy.

On the one hand, I see a real anxiety in many forty-five- to seventy-year-old patients—some feel like walking time bombs, as if their bodies are about to finally reveal cancer, heart disease, lupus, or osteoporosis. Subsequently, there are reports of more eating disorders in older women, more medication use, more depression, adrenal fatigue, and more alcohol consumption.

But on the other hand, I also see women who experience more vitality, better nutrition, and more community. Today there are more books on sex, more yoga practices, more people interested in building stronger bodies and building deeper spiritual connections. Aging during and after menopause is often a time of reckoning—both physical and emotional—but in the wake of its aftermath, many women experience surges of creative energy, confident wisdom, and empowering autonomy. This also can be a time of sexual healing, reignited passions, and intimacy.

Taking all of this into account, how do we prepare ourselves to get through the sexual changes that aging brings?

This also can be a time of sexual healing, reignited passions, and intimacy.

We certainly need a more expansive view of sexual pleasure and sexual pleasuring. Often I see women with teams of sex police or monitors in their heads. Women need to feel empowered to reclaim their sexuality on their own terms and at their own pace. Knowing and exploring oneself is a key step in owning one's pleasure.

If the brain is the most important organ in this regard, then the imagination is the best way to feed it! I regularly suggest that my clients consider sex toys, vibrators, dildos, erotica, or pornography (written or video) to explore new sexual dimensions and new paths to orgasm or sensual pleasure.

It's important to positively reinforce optimal health, happiness, the power of the imagination, and self-acceptance as we age. If joy is the greatest resistance to adversity, this is a call to expand our thoughts and preconceived ideas about sex and pleasure; this pursuit does not have an age limit or a rule book.

FROM THE GOOPASUTRA
LIGHTS ON/LIGHTS OFF

How much time do you now spend on Instagram, Pinterest, and the like? Human beings have always been visual creatures, but our current culture seems to be at an all-time extreme in the visual-stimulation department. We use this information to our detriment at times—negative self-talk and self-consciousness that end in the snapped-off light, the artfully arranged blanket, the tiny skirt tacked onto the bathing-suit bottom.

But we can also use it to our advantage: Humans love seeing other humans—in the flesh. We're *made* to turn each other on. In the context of sex, a live, naked* person has so many advantages over even the most high-definition, beautifully proportioned porn star—we've got pheromones and hormones wildly shooting toward one another in all directions, we've got soft, warm, nothing-like-it-on-earth skin, hair, and lips—it's absolute folly to not deploy our nakedness.

Many of us have body issues; the same mantra that appears elsewhere in this book applies double-time here: "Fake it 'til you make it." No, not everyone wants to leap out of bed and saunter across the room in only their birthday suit, and not everyone wants to leave the lights on and take off their clothes in front of their partner—but do it as often as you can make yourself. You will get positive reinforcement, not just from your partner, but from yourself. Accommodating your body issues' demands at every turn only encourages them; defying them makes sex less self-involved, freer, and more fun.

When the dark becomes a sexy choice instead of a mandate, it, too, becomes more fun.

* *People who sleep naked are said to have way more sex—and enjoy happier relationships overall. There are many studies on the subject (the majority of which seem to be conducted by sheet companies), but common sense also dictates: If you're already naked, it's likelier that one thing will lead to another. Depressing side note: Only 8 percent of Americans are said to sleep naked.*

the holy pelvic floor

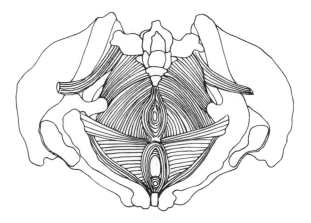

The pelvic floor—the muscle web that acts as a hammock for your undercarriage—sounds like it would be prone to getting stretched out (particularly if you've had kids). But as structural integration and alignment specialist Lauren Roxburgh—author of *Taller, Slimmer, Younger*—explains it, the pelvic floor is one of the body's primary stress containers. When you have a pit in your stomach? That's your pelvic floor in permanent clutch. It's all too easy to lose connection to these muscles—we're not taught how to engage them, and the amount of sitting most of us do doesn't help. Over time, the pelvic floor loses flexibility and tone, which Roxburgh ties to back pain, incontinence—and discomfort during intercourse. Here she shares some simple exercises and tips for regaining strength in your pelvic floor, which she reports is totally possible, and key to great sex.

Strengthening the Pelvic Floor for Better Sex

LAUREN ROXBURGH

What is the pelvic floor?

The pelvic floor is the base of the core. It consists of a sling of muscles that attaches to the bones at the bottom of your pelvis. These muscles effectively form a hammock, or trampoline, across the bottom of your pelvis in two layers: a deep layer and a superficial layer that supports the internal organs above it. Having strong pelvic floor muscles gives you proper control over your bladder and bowels. This can also improve sexual performance and orgasm, help connect you to the deep layers of your core, give your lower back support, help stabilize the hip joints, and act as a lymphatic pump for the pelvis. You get the picture: The pelvic floor muscles are important!

What's the culprit behind pelvic floor issues?

There's actually a pretty simple reason why so many women have issues with incontinence, low back pain, and discomfort in the bedroom. The pelvic floor muscles get stuck and disconnected, and lose tone and elasticity due to sitting too much, tension, and stress.

In Eastern traditions, the pelvic floor area is known as the root chakra—it's where we tend to "hold" fears, specifically fears around primary instincts such as our health, our family's safety, and our financial security. It is a "stress container," in that it's where we process the emotion and house our fight-or-flight reactions. You know that feeling when you get cut off by someone while driving, get bad news, or are about to go into a high-stress situation?

> *You know that feeling when you get cut off by someone while driving, get bad news, or are about to go into a high-stress situation? This can cause you to clench your pelvic floor (it feels like a pit in your stomach) and block energy.*

This can cause you to clench your pelvic floor (it feels like a pit in your stomach) and block energy.

As we hold tension for prolonged periods, it becomes difficult to relax this area, meaning the pelvic floor becomes perma-flexed and rigidly tight. Imagine flexing your biceps constantly and never fully letting go: After a while, this would cause your arm to lose flexibility, strength, tone, and the ability to relax. That's more or less what happens to the pelvic floor until you become aware of the stress and tension and do some work to alleviate it. Part of this work is willfully relaxing and unclenching these muscles—and then directing energy to the region to build strength.

How does the pelvic floor affect a woman's sex life?

Having a strong and flexible pelvic floor is vital to really enjoying sex. This allows you to be in the moment and in your body—not your head—and have more connection around your pelvic floor. Many women feel more confident when they have a toned and resilient pelvic floor; plus, you feel more connected to these muscles, and that can heighten your awareness and sensation during sex. Both these factors help you relax and be more present during sex (great for feeling pleasure and orgasm).

How does having intercourse affect the pelvic floor?

It's a workout for the pelvic floor, and an opportunity to connect to it and really get into your body and feel the amazing energy being exchanged. Try to tune in to the area and practice both contracting and relaxing the pelvic floor while you're having intercourse. It's a great time to do your Kegels (pull in to tighten and hold for about five seconds at a time), which also heightens the sensation for your partner.

Is it always possible to regain strength in the pelvic floor? If so, how?

As with any muscle in the body, yes, in almost every case (barring catastrophic damage to the region), you will be able to regain strength in the pelvic floor. The body has incredible powers to heal when it is treated right and given the optimal exercises to aid in that healing:

Kegels are a great exercise you can do anywhere to help build strength in this region. (I like to squeeze out a set whenever I sit at a red light.)

Pilates is also beneficial, as it's one of the best techniques for working the core (and the pelvic floor is the base of the core).

You can replicate some Pilates moves at home with a foam roller, working the core with a focus on the pelvic floor. Foam rolling is generally a good way to tap into your body and build awareness and coordination of areas like the pelvic floor where you might have lost neuromuscular connection (from the brain to the body).

Last, rebounding (bouncing on a mini trampoline) is another excellent way to build strength and tone in this area. Each time you bounce, you're helping to regenerate strength in the pelvic floor and realign the body.

Simple Pelvic Floor Exercises

THE STRESS ON/OFF BUTTON

To activate your pelvic floor—wherever you are (in the car, on the couch, reading this book)—contract, pull up from the vagina into your core, and hold. You should feel a tightening around your vagina, though try not to tighten your butt or upper belly muscles. Contrast this move by letting go of the muscles: Feel the base of the core relax, and then relax one more layer to fully surrender. If we learn to isolate these muscles with a neuro-muscular or brain-body connection in order to activate and relax them, then we will have better control over how we deal with stress.

GODDESS ROLL

Lie down with your belly facing the mat. Place a foam roller under your hips, with your feet together and knees wide.

Rest your body weight on your forearms, in front of your body.

Keep your belly engaged to prevent overarching your lower back.

Inhale as you slowly roll up to your pubic bone attachment. Keep your upper body still and your forearms on the mat.

Exhale as you roll all the way down to your inner thighs toward your knees. (Again, keeping your upper body still.)

Repeat this movement 8 times.

DEEP SQUATS

This is a basic human movement that we've stopped doing regularly. Getting in the habit of deep squatting will help create proper alignment in the pelvis, lengthen an "uptight" pelvic floor, and increase connection and tone here. It also promotes relief from constipation.

Simply spread your feet wide (mat-width apart) and squat down. Envision going to the bathroom in the woods. For heel support, and if you're on a mat, you can rest your heels on a rolled-up segment of the mat.

Alternatively: Try peeing in the shower squatting down. When you squat to pee, as opposed to sitting up straight on the toilet, you automatically engage your pelvic floor and it naturally stretches, tones, and empties the bladder. Because your urethra is pointed straight down in this position, all you have to do is relax for the urine to flow out easily—as opposed to sitting up straight and having to strain to empty your bladder.

FROM THE GOOPASUTRA
THERE'S AN APP FOR THAT

Besides Kegels, which we always forget to do, one of the easiest ways to work out the pelvic floor that we know of is with the Elvie, an incredibly well-designed and easy to use device-plus-app that takes you through a series of exercises. Here's the deal: You insert a small (smoothly shaped) pod much as you would a tampon. Using Bluetooth, you connect the pod to your phone, and then...you play some games. A session lasts for about five minutes, during which you contract and relax your pelvic floor muscles while watching your progress on-screen, in real time, as your pelvic floor activity effectively moves bars and dots across the screen as directed. Your Elvie workouts are personalized according to your baseline strength (which the app tests for), and the objectives of the exercises vary, increasing in intensity as you go up in levels. (The pulse exercise, FYI, is no joke.)

CHAPTER 35

sexual trauma and the body

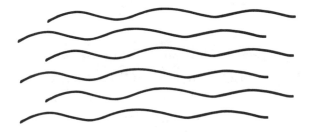

I t goes without saying that healing from sexual trauma is beyond
the scope of this book. At the same time, it's all too common—and
critical—to ignore. A summary by the World Health Organization cited
that about 20 percent of women and between 5 and 10 percent of men
report being victims of sexual violence as children. A national survey covered by the Centers for Disease Control found that nearly the
same percentage of women (1 in 5) report having suffered rape at some
point.

Stephen Porges is a Distinguished University Scientist with the
Kinsey Institute at Indiana University—where his work combines
psychology, neuroscience, and evolutionary biology—and professor
of psychiatry at the University of North Carolina, Chapel Hill. Porges
developed the polyvagal theory, which he uses to examine how the
autonomic nervous system affects the behavior of people who have

experienced trauma. Sexual trauma, Porges has found, becomes locked in the body, suggesting that a way toward healing for many may lie with therapies that focus at least in part on the body.

Unlocking Trauma in the Body

STEPHEN PORGES, PHD

How do you approach the issue of sexual trauma?

Everything has to do with the response of the body. When we use the word "trauma," we don't define it by the event; we define it by the response. This means that for some people, a particular event will be devastating, while others will walk through it.

In terms of health outcomes, it is important to separate the evaluation of the intentionality of the event—which could vary in degree of malevolence in terms of sexual trauma—from the individual's response. From a polyvagal perspective, the individual's response is much more important than the event or the intention of the perpetrator. If we don't emphasize the importance of the individual's response, we may end up blaming and shaming people for their reactions, especially when their responses are disruptive to their ability to regulate their body state, when others appear to be unaffected by the same events. These reactions are reflexive and not voluntary; they're at the level of the body. Sexual trauma triggers life-threat type responses.

How is sexual trauma different from other forms of trauma?

When investigating health-related concerns, sexual trauma seems to have greater impact than other forms of trauma, probably because it is an intrusion into the individual person's physical *and* psychological space. So the person can't avoid it.

How do the brain and the body process sexual trauma?

This question assumes that brain and body reflect different processing systems. As trauma research has evolved, the distinction between neural regulation of brain and body has been dispelled. Currently we would discuss sexual trauma as being manifest in implicit bodily feelings—which are housed in areas of the brainstem that are influenced by both higher brain structures and the organs and structures of the body. These feelings are distinct from our cognitive awareness

Often following sexual trauma there is a major shift in implicit body memories—because the events are so catastrophic to the individual they're literally erased from their memory.

and our visual images and memories. Often following sexual trauma there is a major shift in implicit body memories—because the events are so catastrophic to the individual they're literally erased from their memory.

The survivor of sexual trauma may not have cognitive awareness of the experience, although their *body* has retained the memory and implicit feeling. Trauma therapies try to create a dynamic interaction between the more diffuse implicit bodily feelings and the more explicit memories with a goal of shifting the client's personal narrative to one of greater self-understanding and self-compassion.

Can you talk about the short-term and long-term effects?

There is variation in the terms used to describe trauma and trauma responses. Researchers and clinicians frequently define trauma in terms of the features of the event. Usually they distinguish between acute and complex trauma. An acute trauma is quite well-defined as a specific event such as rape, car accident, surgery, or the death of a loved one. Acute trauma results in a massive shift in the survivor's ability to regulate behavioral state, especially through social interactions. Following an acute trauma, the survivor is immediately different.

Researchers distinguish acute trauma from more complex trauma: Complex trauma is frequently characterized by constant or chronic abuse. These abuses may occur within a relationship in which the survivor is constantly emotionally or physically abused or psychologically manipulated. The physiology of these two trauma categories is probably different, although both may be expressed with similar diagnostic features. Both acute trauma and complex trauma could be characterized by clinicians as including symptoms of post-traumatic stress disorder, but the actual manifestations in the body may be different.

What are the available treatment options and tools?

There's a disconnect between scientific knowledge and clinical treatment, when it comes to how survivors of sexual trauma are treated. Too many people who have experienced sexual trauma go unwitnessed. What does it mean to be witnessed? Following the trauma, has the survivor been engaged in a conversation during which the focus on the survivor is expressing personal feeling? Has a trusted person asked the survivor to "Tell me how you feel"? This process would allow the survivor's implicit bodily experiences to find a voice and not be suppressed and dissociated from the event. In our society, the reaction is often to turn everything into a legal issue, which would focus, not on feelings, but on documenting the event and gathering evidence to prosecute the perpetrator. As a society, we frequently forget or minimize the importance of witnessing the survivor's reaction. Following sexual trauma, survivors frequently immediately start a defensive strategy that includes dissociating the experience from their conscious awareness. Instead, the survivor needs to be present with another individual and witnessed.

The treatments that appear to be the most successful for survivors of sexual trauma frequently incorporate a physical component (i.e., somatic therapies, body psychotherapies). These treatment models enable the survivor, in a sense, to regain contact, or become present with their body. One of the adaptive functions involved in surviving a traumatic experience, such as rape or severe physical abuse, is dissociation. Dissociation enables the body to become numb, and for the sense of awareness to be blunted as mental images move toward an altered reality from the physical event. Dissociation has profoundly devastating effects and is difficult to treat. Medication frequently does not work. Forms of talk therapy may often lower the threshold for reactivity. Dissociation is a powerful adaptive strategy that may functionally protect the trauma survivor from re-experiencing the trauma. Thus, talking about the trauma may trigger dissociation. Therefore, therapies are moving in a different direction, toward an understanding of implicit bodily reactions, and trying to empower our consciousness to create a different personal narrative in which we are no longer shameful of bodily reactions, but understand them as neurobiological adaptations.

Can you explain polyvagal theory and how it relates?

Polyvagal theory emphasizes that the way we react to the world is a function of our physiological state. This is important in dealing with people who have experienced sexual trauma. If survivors of sexual trauma shut down, or go into dissociative withdrawing, their physiological state changes. Their autonomic nervous system changes in the way it regulates the organs of the body. In this changed state, the survivor's perspective of the world is very biased. From a polyvagal perspective, the trauma-induced shift in physiological state results in trauma survivors seeing virtually everyone as a threat. The clinical histories of survivors of sexual violence frequently indicate that they want to have relationships, but they find it hard to be trusting and become intimate. Their bodies won't allow proximity and pleasurable physical contact. Polyvagal theory explains the biobehavioral, the physiological, and the psychological experiences that follow traumatic events. Polyvagal theory also provides clues to reverse these debilitating features. It does this by focusing on strategies to shift the physiological state to enable the individual to be calm and to feel safe.

CHAPTER 36

when you think something may be wrong

The lines between a sexual concern, a disorder, and a dysfunction are typically drawn depending on the severity of the impact on a person's life. But the bottom line is that we should always feel empowered to seek help and answers when any piece of our health (be it sexual, reproductive, or otherwise) is bothering us at all.

Sharon Parish is a professor of medicine in clinical psychiatry and in clinical medicine at Weill Cornell Medical College, Director of Medical Services at New York-Presbyterian Westchester Division, and an attending physician at New York–Presbyterian Hospital in New York City. She splits her NYC practice between general internal medicine and specialized consultations on sexual health. The most common things people come to her with are sexual concerns and questions, particularly around low desire, pain, and arousal difficulty (or at least perceived difficulty). Parish sometimes finds that patients benefit from additional information (i.e., learning that they might need clitoral stimulation to orgasm and what that could look like), or counseling on a life issue that's entwined with their sexuality; and sometimes she suggests more advanced medical intervention. Here, she breaks down what she sees as potentially viable treatment paths for the sexual issues she sees most often.

Common Sexual Concerns, Questions, and Disorders— and How to Get Help

SHARON PARISH, MD

How do you define a sexual disorder?
The most common issues that people come to me for are sexual concerns and questions. Either it's a change of their sexual function with age, or with medication, or with life cycle or relationship status; or they're in a long-term relationship and their desire is different. The question is: Is there a disorder, or is there just a need for sexual information or for counseling?

A sexual disorder is a problem like low desire, low arousal, orgasm difficulties, or sexual pain. Those basic categories of sexual dysfunction follow the Masters and Johnson sexual response cycle, modified by Kaplan and Lief: desire, arousal, and orgasm (there are additional subsets of problems within these categories). A sexual disorder could affect a relationship, quality of life, or cause the person emotional distress or upset—the resulting impact is the distinction between a sexual concern or issue and a disorder. And a disorder becomes a dysfunction, in my opinion, when it causes significant persistent life impairment or distress, either in quality of life, in function, or in a relationship.

What are the most common concerns and disorders you see?

The most common concerns relate to whether stimulation patterns are normal or not. I'll hear: "Sometimes I need to do X, Y, or Z...Why do I only have orgasms with clitoral stimulation?" Or, "Why can't I have orgasms with intercourse?" The solution might be education, learning how some women have orgasms only with clitoral stimulation, and learning techniques for sexual stimulation.

Sometimes the problem is pain with sexual activity, particularly as women get older—when transitioning from menopause to postmenopause as vaginal lubrication declines. Younger women may have pain as well, and low desire is due to the fact they're in pain.

(Good initial web resources include the professional websites of the North American Menopause Society and the International Society for the Study of Women's Sexual Health, and the consumer website MiddlesexMD.)

When is low desire a disorder?

*Hypo*active, meaning low sexual desire, is a distressing loss of sexual desire that impacts either one's intrapersonal happiness or interpersonal relationships and overall function. This kind of lack of desire doesn't respond to lighting a candle, or having a glass of wine, or taking a vacation.

> *This kind of lack of desire doesn't respond to lighting a candle, or having a glass of wine, or taking a vacation.*

It seems to have to do with the brain pathways—whether that's through experience or maybe some kind of biologic predisposition—or it could be a consequence of another medical condition like depression, thyroid problems, or hormonal issues.

What are viable treatment options?

First, it's important to assess and talk with your doctor about the issue you're having and how you're approaching sex in your life. Sometimes it is enough to begin to direct attention to the issue and the patient will solve it on her own. Sometimes it's a lifestyle issue and the patient needs counseling or to take a break from the stressors of daily life. Maybe she isn't getting enough sleep, has too much on her mind, or isn't making sex a priority; or a couple isn't making time in their relationship for sex. The next level of intervention might be referral to a specialist who does sex therapy, mindfulness therapy, or cognitive behavioral therapy—helping the patient or the couple to refocus on the sexual repertoire; or there may even be a need for specific sex therapy that works on technique. Then there are medical interventions where you address modifiable risk factors, for example, treating a hormonal problem or depression.

Along with basic counseling, lifestyle techniques, and sex therapy, very specific education is sometimes needed; for instance, learning when a vibrator or other clitoral stimulators or sex adjuncts (some look like sex toys but are sold as medical treatments) can be helpful. There's a wearable clitoral stimulation device called Fiera, which is designed to be used during foreplay, that helps enhance arousal.

Depending on the patient's symptoms, and if the symptoms are not due to a psychological factor for which basic counseling on lifestyle or relationship therapy could be helpful—or the patient isn't depressed, or switching around their hormonal contraceptive—a doctor might then recommend a prescription drug. There is now an FDA-approved medication, Addyi, for generalized, persistent, distressing low sexual desire in premenopausal women. Addyi's mechanism of action is to balance brain neurotransmitters such that the effect is pro-sexual.

Are there certain genes or lifestyle factors that put you more at risk for sexual disorders?

There's a lot of debate about that. It's clear that there are genetic differences in women who experience depression and those who don't, especially when the depression occurs at an earlier age. But the genetics behind sexual function and responsiveness are still in the very early stages of research. What we do know is that there are differences in responses to treatment that are probably genetically driven.

Some women may be genetically prone to having hypoactive sexual desire, which is actually a disorder or a dysfunction if it impairs life. There is also some theory and evidence that low desire can be imprinted by the neuroplasticity of experience. In other words, having a distressing relationship, or experiencing a period of time when your desire is low, may actually imprint that pathway in your brain. There is still more research being done in these areas.

Lifestyle factors—like relationship issues, psychosocial stressors, medication, substance use, alcohol, opiates, and chronic use of benzodiazepines all seem to affect the brain pathways related to desire.

What's the relationship between alcohol and sexual dysfunction?

In low doses, alcohol causes disinhibition, but in higher doses, it seems to suppress desire and sexual response. This effect is more clear-cut in men, but alcohol, especially heavy use, may have a negative effect on desire and other aspects of sexual function for men and women. If you have a serious drinking problem, too much consumption can eventually cause nerve damage—alcohol is a nerve toxin—which will affect sexual responsiveness.

What should you do if you suspect your partner has a disorder?

Gently bring it up. Don't start with "I think you have a sexual dysfunction." Raise the question in the context of making the relationship better. Say that intimacy and sex are really important in your relationship, and you feel things could be different, or you'd like to explore how to improve it, make it better, or enhance it. Or say that there are concerns you have, and you wonder if your partner would be willing to seek information about them. Encourage them to see their own doctor, or go with them, as appropriate.

treating vaginal dryness

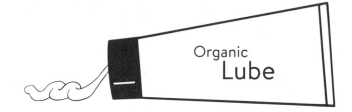

No need to beat around the bush—vaginal dryness is unpleasant. As always, check in with your gynecologist to see if anything more is up. For lubricant options, remedies, and supplement suggestions, we turn back to hormone expert (see her Q&A on hormonal balance on pages 211–222), author of *Younger* (among others) and functional gynecologist Sara Gottfried.

Lubing Up

SARA GOTTFRIED, MD

Vaginal dryness is a common condition for many women. If you are on the pill, you're 25 percent more likely to have vaginal dryness. Another major cause is being postparturm, perimenopausal, or menopausal, due to the withdrawal of estrogen and testosterone in a condition now termed "genitourinary syndrome of menopause." Whether from age or the pill, the vagina can degenerate as estrogen and/or testosterone decrease (yes, women need testosterone, too), which leads to less lubrication and burning, itching, irritation, even pain.

Genitourinary syndrome of menopause, or vaginal atrophy, occurs in up to 50 percent of perimenopausal or menopausal women. That's more than 24 million women in the United States alone and likely is an underestimate because doctors typically don't ask about it.

To treat vaginal dryness, first have a conversation with your gynecologist to rule out any serious concerns. (Rest assured, they will not be embarrassed by whatever you ask.) Since vaginal atrophy can worsen over time, it's best to report your symptoms as soon as possible to get the proper help.

Once you've ruled out any other serious issues, check out one of the many natural ways to lubricate your lady parts and remedy vaginal dryness or atrophy. Here are several options:

1. **Low-dose vaginal estrogen or other estrogen creams:** This is usually the go-to remedy for vaginal dryness. According to research, clinical effects can be excellent, with little to no side effects. Apply using your finger (not the applicator, which shoots the creams too high up for estrogen reception). Use 1 gram of the cream on the outside of the vagina, the inner vaginal lips, clitoris, and opening to the vagina. Apply another 1 gram to the lower third of the vagina.

2. **Hormone-free vaginal moisturizers or lubricants:** For those concerned about using hormonal treatments, hormone-free options include vaginal moisturizers, such as Replens, or vaginal lubricants. Use these products liberally for the full effect. But be aware that they merely alleviate the symptoms short-term.

3. **Vaginal DHEA:** In comparison with estrogens, the hormone DHEA seems to penetrate deeper into the vaginal wall, facilitating healing.

4. **Dietary phytoestrogens:** Studies have shown that phytoestrogens—lower-dose estrogens found in foods or herbs— can improve vaginal dryness. Foods rich in phytoestrogens

include flaxseed, flaxseed oil, and whole organic soy (tofu, miso, tempeh—be sure to avoid GMOs in soy).

I recommend four supplements for vaginal dryness:

1. **Maca:** This dietary supplement has been shown to raise estradiol levels in menopausal women and help with vaginal dryness, as well as depression, memory, concentration, and energy. The recommended dose is 2,000 mg per day, and it comes in powder form. Sprinkle it into smoothies, yogurts, or puddings.
2. **Vitamin E:** This supplement has been shown to increase blood supply to the vaginal wall and improve menopausal symptoms. Doses of 50–400 IU per day are recommended. Don't give up too soon—it might be a month or longer before you feel its effects.
3. **Vitamin D:** This supplement decreases the vaginal pH and dryness associated with vaginal atrophy.
4. **Probiotics:** Researchers have found that vaginal bacterial makeup varies according to a woman's reproductive stage. Therefore, personalized probiotics could be helpful in tackling vaginal atrophy.

FROM THE GOOPASUTRA

NEWER OPTIONS WITH PLEASURE POTENTIAL

Based on dermatologic treatments originally developed for the face, laser treatments for the vagina may help make sex possible for people for whom it's become too painful, and better for those who don't enjoy it as much as they could. The treatments don't hurt; they usually take about ten minutes, and involve no hormones, drugs, or surgery. And their very existence is throwing light onto common yet unspoken problems experienced by women all over the world.

They aren't cheap, there's typically a four-day, no-sex downtime after a session, and much of the technology is so new that there are fewer scientific studies completed than most gynecologists would like. With seemingly positive anecdotal evidence, some gynecologists are already using lasers with their day-to-day patients. At the time of printing, Dr. Gottfried noted that there are no randomized trials published yet proving that lasers are better than the treatments she currently prescribes (which is the standard she requires in order to recommend a treatment to patients). She explains more, and also points to a different research-backed option:

"Some women find that laser therapy—or selective estrogen receptor modulators (SERMs), such as ospemifene—may be helpful for genitourinary syndrome of menopause.[1] SERMs are designed for women with genitourinary syndrome who are at significant risk of breast cancer, and ospemifene is structurally similar to tamoxifen, a prescription therapy for the prevention of breast cancer, but with a full estrogen effect on genitourinary tissues and randomized trials proving safety and effectiveness.[2] In the future, laser therapy may be supported by multiple randomized trials." (Again, and as always, talk to your doctor about what's right for you.)

Notes

1. Arunkalaivanan A et al. "Laser therapy as a treatment modality for genitourinary syndrome of menopause: a critical appraisal of evidence." *International Urogynecology Journal* 2017; 28(5):681–685. doi: 10.1007/s00192-017-3282-y. Epub 2017 Feb 2. https://www.ncbi.nlm.nih.gov/pubmed/28154914; Faubion SS et al. "Genitourinary Syndrome of Menopause: Management Strategies for the Clinician. *Mayo Clin Proceedings* 2017; 92(12):1842–1849. doi: 10.1016/j.mayocp.2017.08.019. https://

www.ncbi.nlm.nih.gov/pubmed/29202940; Kagan R, Rivera E. "Restoring vaginal function in postmenopausal women with genitourinary syndrome of menopause." *Menopause* Sep. 18, 2017. doi: 10.1097/GME.0000000000000958. [Epub ahead of print]. https://www.ncbi.nlm.nih.gov/pubmed/28926510.

2. Pinkerton JV, Kagan R. "Ospemifene for the treatment of postmenopausal vulvar and vaginal atrophy: recommendations for clinical use." *Expert Opinion on Pharmacotherapy* 2015; 16(17):2703–14. doi: 10.1517/14656566.2015.1109627. Epub Dec. 3, 2015. https://www.ncbi.nlm.nih.gov/pubmed/26634778; Wurz, GT et al. "Safety and efficacy of ospemifene for the treatment of dyspareunia associated with vulvar and vaginal atrophy due to menopause." *Clinical Interventions in Aging* 2014; 13;9:1939–50. doi: 10.2147/CIA.S73753. eCollection 2014. https://www.ncbi.nlm.nih.gov/pubmed/25419123; Portman, D et al. "Ospemifene, a non-oestrogen selective oestrogen receptor modulator for the treatment of vaginal dryness associated with postmenopausal vulvar and vaginal atrophy: a randomised, placebo-controlled, phase III trial." *Maturitas* 2014; 78(2):91–98. doi: 10.1016/j.maturitas.2014.02.015. Epub Mar. 12, 2014. https://www.ncbi.nlm.nih.gov/pubmed/24679891; DeGregorio MW et al. "Ospemifene: a first-in-class, non-hormonal selective estrogen receptor modulator approved for the treatment of dyspareunia associated with vulvar and vaginal atrophy." *Steroids* 2014; 90:82–93. doi: 10.1016/j.steroids.2014.07.012. Epub Aug. 1, 2014. https://www.ncbi.nlm.nih.gov/pubmed/25087944; Bruyniks N et al. "Effect of ospemifene on moderate or severe symptoms of vulvar and vaginal atrophy." *Climacteric* 2016; 19(1):60–5. doi: 10.3109/13697137.2015.1113517. Epub Nov. 19, 2015. https://www.ncbi.nlm.nih.gov/pubmed/26669628.

CHAPTER 38

the health of the prostate

The prostate, which is said to be a pleasure zone for some men, sits below the bladder, roughly between the penis and the anus. It plays a role in the urinary tract system as well as some of the body's reproductive and sexual functions. Dr. Arthur Burnett, an expert in prostate health and erectile dysfunction and penile abnormalities (among other related fields), says there is still a lot we don't know about the prostate, including how exactly it might relate to sexual pleasure.

Burnett is a professor in the urology department at Johns Hopkins University School of Medicine, director of their Basic Science Laboratory in Neurourology, director of the Male Consultation Clinic at Johns Hopkins Hospital, and a clinician-scientist at the James Buchanan Brady Urological Institute. Here, he explains the basics of prostate health and its potential impacts on reproduction, sex, stimulation, and sensation. (Following his interview, if you're curious about experimenting with pleasure around the prostate, see sexuality coach's Layla Martin's tips on page 259.)

How Does the Prostate Relate to Sex?

ARTHUR BURNETT, MD

How does the prostate influence reproductive and overall health?

The prostate is an organ in the body that works with the urinary tract and is involved in some reproductive and sexual functions. Located at the base of the bladder, it provides almost a course for accessory reproductive tract structures to come through it, like the ejaculatory duct and a variety of the secretory glands. The prostate plays a role in the lubrication of the urethra, providing secretions that help carry the ejaculate and sperm. The prostate circles the urethra so urine runs through it, and some have postulated that it serves a filter function for organisms that may traverse the open end of the urethra and could otherwise get into the body. (This could in part explain what goes wrong in prostatitis, when the gland swells.)

The prostate can become cancerous and is sometimes removed completely; men can survive without the organ and it doesn't typically affect longevity, but its removal can change aspects of bodily function. For instance, without a prostate, the way a person's ejaculatory fluid and sperm traverse can change, so that men who have undergone radical prostatectomies might not be able to conceive naturally.

What are the early warning signs of prostate dysfunction?

It varies depending on the kind of dysfunction:

Prostatitis is an acute infection, or inflammation, of the prostate. This usually involves discomfort between the scrotal and anal areas, and it can flare up to the point that the patient can't sit, experiences burning with urination, and feels extremely achy in that part of the body.

Another is benign prostatic enlargement (BPE), sometimes called the big prostate phenomenon. The prostate enlarges with age (this may relate to changing hormones), which isn't necessarily a problem, but in some cases, an enlarged prostate causes urinary dysfunction by obstructing the urethra. Symptoms include a slow stream, feeling hesitant to urinate, dribbling, increased frequency and urgency, and nighttime urination (called nocturia).

The other major related dysfunction is prostate cancer, which can spread to other areas of the body, as with any other cancer. Early symptoms are nonexistent with prostate cancer. As the prostate gland gets overtaken and the cancer grows, the overgrowth of tissue can obstruct urination and cause rectal problems, as well as a lot of bleeding and pain.

If the diagnosis is early enough, we sometimes offer surgery to remove the prostate or radiation. If the cancer has spread throughout the body, we talk about hormone suppression, or some chemotherapies that are starting to be developed.

What's the link between the prostate and sexual pleasure (and dysfunction)?

The prostate is situated where a lot of the nerves in the deep pelvis course around it and run into the root of the penis, which affects how erections occur due to blood flow. In terms of sexual pleasure, I think the link is still a little more nebulous. Most men can experience sexual stimulation and orgasm sensations even without a prostate, once their erections become functional again—sometimes the nerves are damaged and need time to heal and regain this function. So there may be nerves in that area that confer some sort of ability to feel sensations, reflexive stimulations; or maybe some gentlemen find ways of sexual pleasure with stimulus in the adjacent anal area.

What kind of prostate testing, if any, do you recommend?

This is an area of great debate, particularly within the framework of prostate cancer. Prostate-specific antigen (PSA) testing is a blood test that measures the amount of a protein produced by the prostate—abnormal levels suggest that something is going wrong (potentially prostatitis, BPE, or prostate cancer). Typically, men are screened between the ages of fifty and sixty-five. It's not clear that there's benefit to screening people younger or older. It's recommended that high-risk groups, which include African American men and men with a family history of prostate cancer, get PSA testing much more routinely.

What factors—such as genetics, diet, or lifestyle—affect prostate health?

Which factors are most relevant remains to be fully understood, but there's evidence that a person's genetic makeup may influence their risk of prostate cancer. Similar to cardiovascular health, epidemiological studies suggest that certain lifestyles and behavioral activities affect the health of the prostate. It's generally thought that what is helpful for the heart and the cardiovascular system (like exercise and good nutrition) probably is equivalently beneficial for the prostate; and vice versa—what is detrimental to cardiovascular health is detrimental to the prostate.

FROM THE GOOPASUTRA
A DIFFERENT TAKE ON PROSTATE PLEASURE

As Dr. Burnett points out, the exact link between the prostate and pleasure isn't clear. But some men do seem to derive pleasure from being stimulating in this region. While it takes effort, sexuality coach Layla Martin says it's "so worth it." If you happen to be down, here are her tips:

You can find the prostate by pressing into his perineum—which is the flat area of skin between his balls and his anus—with a thumb or index finger. You can also stroke the prostate up his anus; it is located about 3 to 4 inches inside the anal canal, facing his stomach. Even though this can make some men nervous, once they try it, many describe incredibly intense pleasure and orgasms.

Four keys:

1. Only ever approach the prostate when he is already turned on. If he isn't turned on, touching his prostate will likely feel super uncomfortable.
2. Most men prefer a very firm touch. You can start touching and then ask him if he likes the pressure, but think more intense, not feather light.
3. If you are pleasuring through his perineum, you want to press in deeply, like one or two inches straight in, and you can rhythmically move your finger in and out while keeping it deep, like pressing a button on and off, really sensually. This works best while giving him a hand or blow job.
4. It can be super erotic to stroke the prostate through his anus. Clean your hands, clip your nails, and make sure he's into it first. Once he's turned on, slide a finger into his anus and feel for something around the size of a walnut, or the side of a plum—it sticks out just slightly, about three to four inches inside the anal canal. You can stroke it up and down with your finger, with relatively firm pressure.

CHAPTER 39

sex addiction: what's behind the label?

S ex researchers, clinicians, and the public have different ideas about what constitutes a sex addiction—or even if there is such a thing. We are extremely compelled by the perspective of licensed marriage and family therapists and certified sex therapists Douglas Braun-Harvey and Michael Vigorito, who outline their approach to other clinicians in *Treating Out of Control Sexual Behavior: Rethinking Sex Addiction*. As Braun-Harvey and Vigorito explained to us, they use the term "out of control sexual behavior (OCSB)," as descriptive of someone's subjective experience: "It doesn't mean that they *are* out of control; feelings are different from behavior." What Braun-Harvey and Vigorito try to determine in their assessment of clients is what underlies the behavior, including any source of internal conflict that might add to the sense of being out of control—and what kind of help clients might need to follow through on the changes they want to make. The duo's larger perspective on what's lacking when it comes to men's sexual health, beyond any debate over sex addiction, is enlightening as well.

Understanding Out of Control Sexual Behavior

DOUGLAS BRAUN-HARVEY AND MICHAEL VIGORITO

How is sex addiction defined?

There is no standard definition of sex addiction—you'll get a different definition depending on the theorist you're working with.

Another way of thinking about it is that we're being asked to define Kleenex (a brand), rather than tissues. When we say "sex addiction," we're really talking about a brand, or a label, a conclusory evaluation about a human behavior—rather than using language that invites us to discuss, and be interested in, what the human behavior is. We should be asking: How do we understand human behavior when people's sexual behavior feels out of their control?

When clients come to us and self-identify as "sex addicts" or describe their behavior as addictive or compulsive, it's our job as clinicians to remain curious about the underlying issues. If a patient goes to a doctor and says, "I have cancer," the doctor won't say, "Now I don't have to go and run all those tests. Let's start treatment."

As clinicians, we want to evaluate the client's sexual behavior concern assessment so we can better understand what's happening with them.

Where did the term "out of control sexual behavior" originate?

In 2004, Dr. John Bancroft, the eminent sex researcher from the United Kingdom, published a journal article recommending use of the phrase "out of control sexual behavior (OCSB)" rather than the term "sex addiction" until we had a scientific consensus and understood exactly what we were talking about. He liked the term OCSB because it was not evaluative. It describes what a person is going through, what they feel and experience, rather than being a diagnosis, or inserting diagnostic-sounding labels.

We define OCSB as a sexual health problem in which a person's consensual sexual urges, thoughts, or behaviors feel out of control. We don't say: "Look, you're doing this thing, that must be out of control; you're out of control." We hear the term "sex addiction" or "sexual compulsivity" as a metaphor for someone telling us that there are times when they feel out of control, and they are now asking for help around that issue.

What are out of control sexual behaviors?

Let's first exclude what we don't consider OCSB, which differs from other models, particularly sex addiction. The sex addiction model includes nonconsensual, predatory sexual behavior, and sexual harassment. The OCSB model excludes nonconsensual behavior. If somebody is involved in violations of somebody else's body, forced sex—that's an entirely different issue. People engaging in nonconsensual sex should have treatment from experts who specialize in that, so this is one of the first things we screen for.

We screen for other factors as well. We have to make sure the person isn't abusing drugs or alcohol in a way that affects their sexual behavior; isn't living amid extreme violence (e.g., intimate partner violence); and does not have an untreated mental health issue, physical condition, or a medication side effect. We want to make sure these things aren't the explanation for OCSB before starting treatment.

Typically, with men who are saying, "I feel out of control," this is what we see: There's a contradiction between how they act and they would like to act. For instance, they're not keeping the agreements they have in relationships with their partners. Or they are not keeping agreements with themselves—their sexual behavior contradicts their personal values or what they consider to be appropriate sexual behavior for themselves. There can be exploitative, deceptive behavior in the clients we work with, where they're trying to present, or act, in one way, yet they're behaving in a contradictory way.

Often, their concerns are looking at sexual imagery when they masturbate or extramarital/extrarelational sexual behavior outside the agreements of that relationship. Others are concerned about paying for sex, or repeatedly engaging in high-risk sexual behaviors.

How do you assess a client?

The first meeting is a consultation where we want to understand the precipitating event that brought them into therapy. We screen for the vulnerability factors just outlined, and determine if there's another treatment priority (e.g., drug rehabilitation). We want to understand why they are here (aka their motivation)—which should not be just because their spouse or their church sent them—sustained change occurs when the reason for change comes from them.

We recommend a comprehensive assessment; it can be four to eight individual sessions, sometimes more. We conduct a clinical evaluation to examine all the ways their sexual health could be disrupted. (For instance, they may have a secret sexual turn-on they are afraid to tell their partner and the secret-keeping feels out of control; or they have a really high sex drive and are struggling to manage.) At the end, we review their clinical picture in a way that hopefully isn't a surprise to them, because we've been talking with them, raising their awareness, the whole time. From there, we develop their sexual health plan.

What does treatment entail?

For the people we think could benefit from treatment for OCSB, we recommend weekly group therapy, alongside supportive individual therapy (no less than once every six weeks). We might also refer a patient to a psychiatrist, or a couples therapist, and create a community treatment team to address and achieve their sexual health goals.

There are three areas we work on in therapy:

1. **How men regulate their behaviors.** We teach skills and ways to become better regulators, using a realm of psychology and research on self-regulation and coregulation (how we regulate ourselves through relationships with others) involving the environment, internal systems, the body, and the mind.

2. **Relationships and attachment.** How do men get close to people? How do they create distance when they need it? Oftentimes, the sexual behavior has been a way to create closeness and distance, without having to create closeness and distance in more functional, direct, and honest ways.

3. **Erotic conflict.** Almost all standard methods are poor at treating this area. People are conflicted about what arouses them, what excites them, what interests them sexually, what turns them on. Some people, men in particular, are more prone to have what are typically called paraphilias or fetishes, or very fixed turn-ons. Some men have never come to terms with the fact that they have these kinds of turn-ons. They're ashamed of them, and handle them in ways that cause hurt and injury. Anytime you are at war with a part of yourself, you're not going to regulate yourself very well. We find that a fairly significant percentage of men who feel out of control with sexual behavior have just not made peace with their erotic nature.

What should you do if you feel your partner has an out of control sex behavior?

Don't jump to conclusions and try to self-diagnose the situation. Call a certified sex therapist or a couples therapist with experience addressing sexuality, and go together for an appointment. Have a space where you can talk about this openly with someone who is trained to discuss sexual matters without making assumptions about what's going on. Often what a partner does is call a sex addiction therapist, or somebody who works with spouses of sex addicts, but then you've already determined what the problem is by consulting a "specialist" before going to an expert who is more likely to first look at the bigger picture. (Also, it's important to know that you can become a "certified sex addiction therapist" in the United States and not have to take a single course on sexuality. Someone who is certified to do sex addiction therapy does not need to have the same level of training and knowledge in sexuality as a certified sex therapist.)

Do you find that people often pretend to have a sex addiction?

In the storm of betrayal, a client is often still motivated to maintain the relationship, even though their behavior has hurt the person they love. They might feel intense shame and guilt, and may label their behavior "sex addiction" as a way to provide a map for understanding what's been happening, or as hope that they can salvage the relationship. It might give them time to seek treatment.

There are very expensive inpatient treatment programs for sex addiction around the country, where patients pay $50,000, even $100,000 per program. If people have the money and the wherewithal, they might go to these programs as a way to demonstrate to a partner that they're very remorseful and committed to change. Does that mean they have a sex addiction? Or that they need that level of treatment? Not necessarily.

Is infidelity ever an OCSB?

We don't see OCSB as a diagnosis or disorder, and we're not really interested in if there's a sexual disorder. If the person believes they have a problem, we're more interested in determining what kind of change they want to make, and what level of help might be beneficial for them. We help people think of behaviors as having functions. So, what problem was that sexual behavior trying to solve? In therapy, people can begin to understand why they made the choices they made, even though their decisions hurt people. We want to help people who feel out of control come up with better plans to address the problems they're having.

Why do you work only with men?

The mental health field doesn't have a good track record when it comes to sorting out distinctions between sexual problems and basic prejudices. If you look back to the 1960s, when the birth control pill came out, there was a concern of women becoming "out of control" sexually. Called nymphomania, this was a real diagnosis, and the belief was that if women didn't have to be afraid of pregnancy, they would have no reason to control themselves sexually.

We've encouraged other professionals to develop treatments that could be specifically helpful to women. There are so many biases inherent in the definition of OCSB that you would need a good, gender-informed model for treating women for OCSB (which we haven't seen yet), so that it would not be overly informed by gender bias and stereotypes against women who are not conforming to sexual standards. Women face many different consequences for not conforming to sexual standards that men don't.

Women face many different consequences for not conforming to sexual standards that men don't.

Also, women aren't coming forward in any kind of the percentages that men are and saying they have out of control sexual behavior.

What do men specifically struggle with as it relates to sexual health?

Culturally, how do we teach men to get their sexual needs met? We don't necessarily prepare men to manage the tension between pleasure and safety, or socialize men to be open and honest about what they like sexually or what they find pleasurable in romantic relationships. As a society, we are not very interested in helping men with their sexual health until after someone has been hurt.

Men don't have many places to talk about or understand who they are sexually. Often, they're literally watching sexual entertainment to understand who they are sexually and educate themselves. (Which would be like going to a war movie to learn responsible firearm safety.)

We want to create a space where men can better understand their sexuality, where we can become curious about the binds that they find themselves in sexually, and where we can help them find solutions.

FROM THE GOOPASUTRA
SEX TIPS (AND UN-TIPS)

The GOOPiest sex tip ever might be this (unedited quote): "Drink lots of water—it affects everything." But communication—which nearly every expert we interviewed for the book highlighted—was the strongest recurring theme among staffers. Here's what else makes the list:

- "Don't overthink it. No one is a pro, whether they think so or not. No matter how much experience you have, there is always something new to learn."

- "Presence and enthusiasm are everything. Being present (i.e., clearheaded and detached from judgment) heightens true connection and your ability to respond to and with your partner. Eye contact goes a long way, too."

- "Communicate. Be open about what you what. Our bodies will tell our lovers what we want, but we still aren't mind readers."

- "Trusting the person you're with makes all the difference."

- "Just be free—sex isn't always pretty and natural, so don't worry about looking good all of the time."

- "Always share with your partner exactly what you want (and guide them) during sex. It makes my partner and me so much more aroused when I/he gets to communicate how amazing it feels."

- "Hotel rooms are an aphrodisiac. If the spark needs a little help, plan a little getaway, even if it's just for one night. Note: Bathtub sex is never what it looks like in the movies."

- "Only do something if you're truly into it. Partners can always tell when you're doing something out of obligation."

- "Find the right partner. My current partner is great in bed. Everyone before just wasn't as good and I didn't even know I was missing out on really amazing sex. So I guess, in a way, sleep around?"

- "The more you relax and allow yourself to be present, the more you'll enjoy. Relaxing has to be a conscious choice for us as women, because we sometimes aren't even aware that we're carrying the stresses of work, parenting, finance, etc., with us into the bedroom; it prevents climax and a rewarding sexual experience."

- "Try to shut off your brain to everything else going on. Turn on music, or do whatever helps you get into the zone."

- "Pretend you're a porn star. Get into it, and they will, too."

last thing

By no means a conclusion or a final word—this book was our attempt at continuing some of the conversations we've had with readers, friends, lovers, and an ever-expanding network of experts and leading thinkers; while also opening up to new conversations we'd like to have more of in the future.

As Esther Perel once told us, it's the silencing around sex that can be most damaging: "How can you learn to talk about something that you've learned to be silent on your whole life?" she asks. "How do you know that what you're experiencing is normal if you can never ask the person next to you?"

We hope you'll be a person to chat about sexuality with, an inviting ear behind closed doors, and an advocate for your own sexual health, desires, and the pursuit of pleasure out in the world.

Talk soon.

acknowledgments

Thank you to our experts featured here who challenged our preconceived notions about sex and opened our minds to a much more interesting universe of possibilities. We are so incredibly grateful: Juliet Allen; Amanda Chantal Bacon; Michaela Boehm; Douglas Braun-Harvey; Arthur Burnett; Shannon Chavez; Zelaika S. Hepworth Clarke; Laura Corn; Adam Cunliffe; Nicole Daedone; Chris Donaghue; Eli Finkel; Suzannah Galland; Sara Gottfried; Alexandra Jamieson; Jillian Keenan; Ian Kerner; Justin Lehmiller; Erika Lust; Layla Martin; Barry Michels; Laurie Mintz; Lane Moore; Emily Morse; Maggie Ney; Peggy Orenstein; Sharon Parish; Esther Perel; Stephen Porges; Nicole Prause; Virginia Reath; Shiva Rose; Lauren Roxburgh; Schuyler Samperton; Eric G. Schneider; Susan Stryker; Betony Vernon; Michael Vigorito; and Londin Angel Winters.

Thank you to everyone at Grand Central Life & Style and Hachette for saying yes to pushing boundaries and for turning our desires into a more thoughtful book, especially Karen Murgolo, Ben Sevier, Morgan Hedden, Claire Brown, Amanda Pritzker, Nick Small, Adam Strange, and Nicole Bond.

For all the iconic illustrations, thank you to Christine Mitchell Adams.

A big thanks to everyone at GOOP HQ who shared their funny, sad, bright, thought-provoking, intimate stories and oft-illuminating sex tips with us—both anonymously and not. To our sex book team—Jessie Geoffray, Julie Jen, Jean Godfrey-June, Kiki Koro-shetz, Elise Loehnen, Gwyneth Paltrow, Ashley Sargent Price, Jenny Westerhoff—that goes double.

Again (and as always), thanks to our readers, who inspired this book and too much else to list.

index